D1330694

RevMED

300 SBAs in
Medicine and Surgery

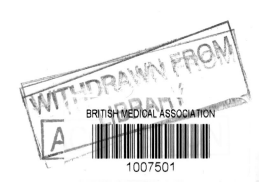

WITHDRAWN FROM LIBRARY

BRITISH MEDICAL ASSOCIATION

A

1007501

Other Related Titles from World Scientific

300 Single Best Answers in Clinical Medicine
by George Collins, James Davis and Oscar Swift
edited by Huw Beynon
ISBN: 978-1-78326-436-0
ISBN: 978-1-78326-437-7 (pbk)

320 Single Best Answer Questions for Final Year Medical Students
by Adam Ioannou
ISBN: 978-981-3146-37-2
ISBN: 978-981-3146-38-9 (pbk)

The PICU Book: A Primer for Medical Students, Residents and Acute Care Practitioners
edited by Ronald M Perkin, Irma Fiordalisi and William E Novotny
ISBN: 978-981-4329-60-6

Surgical Talk: Lecture Notes in Undergraduate Surgery
3rd Edition
by Andrew Goldberg and Gerard Stansby
ISBN: 978-1-84816-614-1 (pbk)

RevMED

300 SBAs in
Medicine and Surgery

Lasith Ranasinghe • Oliver Clements

Imperial College London, UK

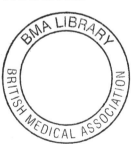

BMA LIBRARY
BRITISH MEDICAL ASSOCIATION

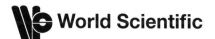 **World Scientific**

NEW JERSEY · LONDON · SINGAPORE · BEIJING · SHANGHAI · HONG KONG · TAIPEI · CHENNAI · TOKYO

Published by

World Scientific Publishing Europe Ltd.

57 Shelton Street, Covent Garden, London WC2H 9HE

Head office: 5 Toh Tuck Link, Singapore 596224

USA office: 27 Warren Street, Suite 401-402, Hackensack, NJ 07601

Library of Congress Cataloging-in-Publication Data

Names: Ranasinghe, Lasith, author. | Clements, Oliver, author.

Title: RevMED : 300 SBAs in medicine and surgery / Lasith Ranasinghe
(Imperial College London, UK) and Oliver Clements (Imperial College London, UK).

Other titles: 300 single best answers in medicine and surgery | Three hundred SBAs in
medicine and surgery

Description: New Jersey : World Scientific, 2019. | Includes index.

Identifiers: LCCN 2018060370| ISBN 9781786346810 (hardback : alk. paper) |
ISBN 9781786347114 (paperback : alk. paper)

Subjects: | MESH: Clinical Medicine--education | Education, Medical--methods |
Examination Question | Case Reports

Classification: LCC RC58 | NLM WB 18.2 | DDC 616.0076--dc23

LC record available at https://lccn.loc.gov/2018060370

British Library Cataloguing-in-Publication Data

A catalogue record for this book is available from the British Library.

Copyright © 2019 by World Scientific Publishing Europe Ltd.

*All rights reserved. This book, or parts thereof, may not be reproduced in any form or by any means,
electronic or mechanical, including photocopying, recording or any information storage and retrieval
system now known or to be invented, without written permission from the Publisher.*

For photocopying of material in this volume, please pay a copying fee through the Copyright Clearance
Center, Inc., 222 Rosewood Drive, Danvers, MA 01923, USA. In this case permission to photocopy
is not required from the publisher.

For any available supplementary material, please visit
https://www.worldscientific.com/worldscibooks/10.1142/Q0203#t=suppl

Desk Editors: Aanand Jayaraman/Jennifer Brough/Shi Ying Koe

Typeset by Stallion Press
Email: enquiries@stallionpress.com

Printed in Singapore by Mainland Press Pte Ltd.

To my niece, Ayana, for the motivation,
to my brother and sister-in-law for their constant support,
and to my parents for providing me with a life that
made my achievements possible.

— Lasith Ranasinghe

For my mum and partner, Ros.
This project would not have been possible
without your unconditional love, support
and encouragement.

— Oliver Clements

Foreword

After 25 years as a doctor, it is nice to be able to say that in all honesty, if I had my time again, I would do exactly the same. Medicine is difficult, as is any high-level career, but I have a truly fascinating job, wonderful friends and colleagues, and make a good living. Moreover, I am far from bored and still have plenty to learn. Medicine commits you to life-long learning and teaching. This publication is very much in this spirit, produced by medical students and doctors, wholly clinical and applicable to everyday medicine, while aiding the passage of students through to qualification. Good luck and I hope you can say the same in another 25 years!

Dr. Jonathan Hoare
Consultant Gastroenterologist
Honorary President of the Imperial College
School of Medicine Medical Education Society

Preface

Single best answer (SBA) questions are a popular examination format that is used at most medical schools across the world. It tests the ability of students to assess a clinical situation, consider the options available and decide on a suitable option; much like real-life clinical practice. This book was written whilst we were preparing for our written clinical exams at Imperial College London. Having used several question books during revision, we became aware of the pros and cons of each book and we developed a vision of what makes the 'ideal' SBA book. This motivated us to take our experiences into account and design our own SBA book.

The current paradigm amongst most medical students is that SBAs are useful for 'testing' knowledge once you have gone through the lectures and textbooks. However, SBAs can, in fact, prove to be a powerful 'learning' tool. Even if you are not particularly confident in your medical knowledge, I implore you to attempt some of these questions. By, firstly, engaging with the question and then studying the explanation, you will, in effect, be taking part in an interactive case-based tutorial that teaches an important concept in medicine. Having the SBA attached to the concept helps cement the knowledge in a more enjoyable and effective way than wading through bland blocks of text in textbooks.

We hope that the questions and explanations in this book will aid your learning as well as improving your exam technique during the revision period. It is designed with the needs and preferences of medical students in mind, so we sincerely hope that you take a liking to the content and format. We wish you all the best for your clinical exams!

Lasith Ranasinghe and Oliver Clements
Imperial College School of Medicine

About the Authors

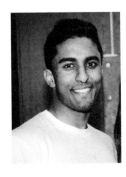 **Lasith Ranasinghe** is a 5th year Medical Student at Imperial College School of Medicine. He grew up in Norwich before starting Medicine at Imperial College London in 2014. He developed an interest in medical education having delivered several lectures to younger students, co-chairing the Medical Education (MedED) society and undertaking the role of Academic Officer of the Students' Union. He has maintained a high academic reputation for having been placed consistently in the top 10 among his cohort and achieving three prizes for academic excellence. He recently completed his BSc in Pharmacology with a First Class (Hons). In his spare time, he runs a charity, 'Smile', which raises money to improve the standard of education for underprivileged children in Sri Lanka. He also enjoys playing football and cricket for ICSM FC and IMCC, respectively.

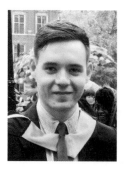

Oliver Clements is a 5th year Medical Student at Imperial College School of Medicine. Originally from High Wycombe, he was the only student from his secondary school to gain admission into a medical school. During his time at Imperial College London, he involved himself in educational initiatives, such as organising tutorials for younger students. His teaching background extends beyond medical school, having tutored Science and Maths at GCSE- and A-level. He maintains a high reputation at medical school, having achieved merits in the 1st and 2nd year. He recently completed his BSc in Gastroenterology and Hepatology with a First Class (Hons) and also presented his project at an international conference and won the Naranjan Singh Virdee Prize for his exceptional cholangiocarcinoma research. In his spare time, he enjoys playing football, cross-country running and fitness.

About the Reviewers

Dr. Sukhpreet Singh Dubb — Alumnus of Imperial College School of Medicine.

Prof. Karim Meeran — Professor of Endocrinology, Imperial College School of Medicine.

Dr. Phillippe Grunstein — Consultant in Respiratory Medicine, Norfolk and Norwich University Hospital.

Dr. Rohit Chitkara — Management Consultant at PwC, previously Teaching Fellow at Hillingdon Hospital.

Dr. Sadia Khan — Consultant Cardiology, West Middlesex University Hospital.

Dr. Shahid Khan — Consultant Gastroenterologist, St Mary's and Hammersmith Hospitals; Honorary Clinical Senior Lecturer, Adjunct Reader, Imperial College School of Medicine.

Acknowledgements

We would like to thank Catharina Weijman and the staff at World Scientific for handling our book proposal with the greatest enthusiasm and kindness, and we would like to thank Isabelle Nicholls (University of Bristol), George Stannard (University of Oxford), and Ravi De Silva (University College London) for reviewing sample chapters and providing much needed feedback to help fine-tune our book.

Lasith Ranasinghe and Oliver Clements
Imperial College School of Medicine

Contents

Paper 1

Questions

1. A 43-year-old man presents with a painless lump in his groin that appeared 2 weeks ago. He claims that the lump protrudes on defecation and he also reports becoming constipated recently. On examination, the lump is reduced and a finger is placed over the midpoint of the inguinal ligament. When the patient is asked to cough, the lump reappears. What is the most likely diagnosis?

   A Direct inguinal hernia
   B Indirect inguinal hernia
   C Femoral hernia
   D Obturator hernia
   E Spigelian hernia

2. Which of the following murmurs is associated with severe aortic regurgitation?

   A Austin-Flint
   B Graham-Steell
   C Gibson
   D Carey-Coombs
   E Barlow

3. A 67-year-old man is brought into A&E having been involved in a road traffic accident. On examination, he opens his eyes to pain, makes a few grunting noises and withdraws his legs from painful stimuli. What is his GCS?

   A 2
   B 4
   C 6
   D 8
   E 10

4. A 2-year-old boy is brought to the GP after his father noticed some swelling around his eyes. On examination, there is periorbital and pedal oedema. A urine dipstick is positive for proteins and negative for blood. What is the most likely diagnosis?

   A IgA nephropathy
   B Membranous glomerulonephritis
   C Rapidly progressive glomerulonephritis
   D Minimal change glomerulonephritis
   E Henoch–Schönlein purpura

5. A 54-year-old man is brought into A&E with a suspected acute coronary syndrome. An ECG is performed, which reveals ST elevation in leads I, aVL, V5 and V6. Which coronary artery has been occluded?

   A Left main stem
   B Left anterior descending coronary artery
   C Left circumflex coronary artery
   D Right coronary artery
   E Posterior descending artery

6. A 46-year-old housewife visits her GP complaining of pain in the joints of her hands that has gradually got worse over 3 months. It has started affecting her ability to complete daily tasks such as cooking for her children. Both of her hands are affected equally and the pain

and stiffness is worst in the morning but gets better when she starts using her hands. On closer inspection, her hands do not appear to be deformed although her metacarpophalangeal joints and proximal interphalangeal joints appear slightly swollen, warm and tender. What is the most likely diagnosis?

    A Reactive arthritis
    B Osteoarthritis
    C Rheumatoid arthritis
    D Psoriatic arthritis
    E Septic arthritis

7. A 56-year-old man with a history of alcoholism complains of intermittent epigastric pain that radiates through to his back. When questioned, he admits to losing about 3 kg in weight over the past 6 months and says that his stools have become pale and difficult to flush away. Which investigation would you request to aid the diagnosis?

    A Serum amylase
    B Blood cultures
    C Faecal elastase
    D CA 19-9
    E OGD

8. A 25-year-old female has suffered from shortness of breath over the past 2 months. She gets particularly breathless when she exerts herself, and has had to stop going on her morning jog. She has not experienced a cough, fever or chest pain. She has no past medical history of note, however, her periods have become quite heavy over the past 3 or 4 months. What is the most likely diagnosis?

    A Hyperthyroidism
    B Anaemia
    C Pneumonia
    D COPD
    E Asthma

9. A 46-year-old man, with a history of type-1 diabetes, visits the GP for an HbA1c reading. He has recently been feeling more tired than usual and has noticed that the skin on his hands has become darker over the past few months. On examination, hepatomegaly and a tanned complexion (despite not having been on any recent holidays) are noted. Haemochromatosis is suspected and iron studies are requested. Which set of results would be consistent with haemochromatosis?

   A High serum iron, high ferritin, high transferrin, low transferrin saturation, low TIBC
   B High serum iron, low ferritin, low transferrin, high transferrin saturation, low TIBC
   C High serum iron, high ferritin, high transferrin, high transferrin saturation, low TIBC
   D High serum iron, high ferritin, low transferrin, high transferrin saturation, high TIBC
   E High serum iron, high ferritin, low transferrin, high transferrin saturation, low TIBC

10. A 72-year-old woman has recently suffered a fracture of her right distal radius after falling on an outstretched hand. She is at high risk of osteoporosis because she is post-menopausal and has undergone several decades of steroid treatment for her asthma. A DEXA scan is performed. Which result would be diagnostic of osteoporosis?

   A T-score of −1.5 or worse
   B T-score of −2 or worse
   C T-score of −2.5 or worse
   D T-score of −3 or worse
   E T-score of −3.5 or worse

11. A 52-year-old man was watching TV yesterday when he suddenly become very aware of his heart beating rapidly. This lasted around 45 mins and then subsided spontaneously. It has happened several times over the past 2 months. An ECG reveals no abnormalities. However, due to the strong suspicion of atrial fibrillation, the patient

is placed on a 24-hr tape, which confirms the diagnosis. Which scoring system should be used to determine the benefit of long-term anticoagulation in this patient?

    A QRISK2 score
    B $ABCD^2$ score
    C GRACE score
    D CHA_2DS_2-VASc score
    E CURB-65 score

12. Which of the following is not a feature of background diabetic retinopathy?

    A Hard exudates
    B Cotton wool spots
    C Microaneurysms
    D Blot haemorrhages
    E Leakage of lipids from blood vessels

13. A 53-year-old man, who has recently recovered from a diarrhoeal illness, comes to A&E with a 1-week history of gradually worsening weakness in his legs. A neurological examination reveals reduced tone, reduced reflexes and impaired sensation in both lower limbs. He adds that the weakness began in his feet and has gradually progressed up his legs. Guillain–Barré syndrome is suspected. Which of the following parameters should be closely monitored in this patient?

    A Body temperature
    B Serum osmolality
    C Serum potassium
    D Forced vital capacity
    E Urine output

14. A 14-year-old school boy was diagnosed with asthma 6 months ago. He was given a salbutamol inhaler to use PRN, however, he continued to have regular episodes of breathlessness. He was started on a regular

inhaled corticosteroid (beclomethasone) 3 months ago. Although the frequency of his attacks has reduced with the medication, he is still experiencing bouts of breathlessness about four times per week. What would be the next most appropriate step in his management?

    A Increase the dose of salbutamol
    B Change the inhaled corticosteroid
    C Add an oral corticosteroid
    D Add a long-acting beta agonist
    E Montelukast therapy

15. Which of the following is the most common cause of chronic kidney disease?

    A Hypertension
    B Diabetes mellitus
    C Glomerulonephritis
    D Pyelonephritis
    E Polycystic kidney disease

16. A 46-year-old woman has been suffering from frequent headaches over the past 4 months, along with some blurring of vision. She also mentions that she has developed a fiercely itchy rash on several occasions, usually occurring soon after she has had a bath. What is the most likely diagnosis?

    A Anaemia
    B Acute lymphoblastic leukaemia
    C Chronic myeloid leukaemia
    D Polycythaemia vera
    E Myelofibrosis

17. A 27-year-old female comes to A&E complaining of severe right iliac fossa pain. She has vomited three times whilst waiting to be seen. On examination, there is rebound and percussion tenderness in the

right iliac fossa and the pain gets worse when the doctor extends the patient's hip. What is the name of the sign being elicited?

    A Murphy's sign
    B Obturator sign
    C Rovsing's sign
    D Psoas sign
    E Aarons sign

18. A 74-year-old man presents with a skin lesion on his left cheek, which has gradually grown over 4 months. On closer examination, the lesion has raised, everted edges with an ulcerated centre revealing a keratotic core. What is the most likely diagnosis?

    A Basal cell carcinoma
    B Squamous cell carcinoma
    C Melanoma
    D Keratoacanthoma
    E Actinic keratosis

19. A 53-year-old man presents to A&E with severe pain in his right flank that radiates to his right groin. Ureteric colic is suspected and a CT-KUB is requested. The CT-KUB confirms the diagnosis but it also shows an abdominal aortic aneurysm with a diameter of 4.7 cm. When questioned, the patient denies any back pain (other than the pain caused by ureteric colic) or symptoms of vascular disease. What is the most appropriate management option for this patient?

    A Reassure and discharge
    B Surveillance with an ultrasound scan every 1 year
    C Surveillance with an ultrasound scan every 6 months
    D Surveillance with an ultrasound scan every 3 months
    E Surgical repair of the aneurysm

20. A 38-year-old man is complaining of excessive thirst and frequent urination over the past month. He describes the thirst as being

'insatiable', and claims to drink about 8–12 litres of water every day. He undergoes a water deprivation test, which revealed the following results:

Urine osmolality
2 hrs: 212 mOsm/kg
4 hrs: 227 mOsm/kg
6 hrs: 221 mOsm/kg
8 hrs: 242 mOsm/kg

Following administration of 2 mg IM desmopressin (DDAVP): 278 mOsm/kg (normal > 600 mOsm/kg). What is the most likely diagnosis?

A Diabetes mellitus type 1
B Central diabetes insipidus
C Nephrogenic diabetes insipidus
D Psychogenic polydipsia
E Hyperparathyroidism

21. A 37-year-old man visits the GP because his partner has recently noticed some dark patches on his back. On examination, there are multiple painless red papules on his back, some of which have merged to form purple plaques. He was diagnosed with HIV 8 years ago. What is the most likely diagnosis?

A Discoid lupus
B Guttate psoriasis
C Kaposi's sarcoma
D Shingles
E Chronic mucocutaneous candidiasis

22. A 16-year-old school girl has been suffering from depression for 6 months. Last night (12 hr ago), she decided to end her life and ingested 40 paracetamol tablets. She has since decided that she has made a mistake and does not want to end her life. She appears

reasonably well when she presents to A&E, only complaining of some mild nausea. What is the most appropriate treatment option?

    A N-acetylcysteine
    B Naloxone
    C Flumezanil
    D Atropine
    E Sodium bicarbonate

23. A 7-year-old girl has had severe, bloody diarrhoea with cramping abdominal pain for the past 3 days. She has also been emptying her bladder less and less frequently. Blood tests, including a blood film, are performed which revealed a low Hb, low platelets and the presence of schistocytes. U&Es are also performed:

Creatinine: 182 μmol/L (baseline = 92 μmol/L)
Urea: 9.2 mmol/L (2.5–6.7)
A stool culture identifies *E. coli* O157. What is the most likely diagnosis?

    A Microangiopathic haemolytic anaemia
    B Haemolytic uraemic syndrome
    C Thrombotic thrombocytopaenic purpura
    D Disseminated intravascular coagulation
    E Gastroenteritis

24. A 37-year-old businessman presents to his GP with a week-long history of headache, diarrhoea and fever. Since he returned from a business trip abroad 2 days ago, he has also developed a dry cough and his wife has commented that he has appeared to be quite confused. What is the most appropriate investigation?

    A CT head scan
    B Urinary antigens
    C Stool culture
    D LFTs
    E U&Es

25. Which system is used to stage prostate cancer?

    A Breslow thickness
    B Gleason staging
    C GRACE score
    D Wells score
    E Dukes' staging

26. A 28-year-old woman presents with a 5-day history of urinary frequency, dysuria and mild suprapubic pain. Urine dipstick is positive for nitrites and leucocytes. A urinary tract infection is suspected and an MSU is taken and sent to the lab. Whilst awaiting culture and sensitivities, which empirical treatment option is best for this patient?

    A Trimethoprim
    B Benzylpenicillin
    C Vancomycin
    D Metronidazole
    E Levofloxacin

27. A 68-year-old male visits his GP complaining of constipation, rectal bleeding and itchiness around his anus. He often feels 'a lump' hanging out after defecating which he has to push back in himself. On examination, anal tone is weak and a protruding mass is felt which has palpable muscular rings. What is the most likely diagnosis?

    A Grade 3 haemorrhoids
    B Grade 4 haemorrhoids
    C Perianal abscess
    D Type 1 rectal prolapse
    E Type 2 rectal prolapse

28. A 54-year-old man is complaining of sharp, central chest pain that has arisen over the last 24 hrs. On inspection, the patient is sitting forward on the examination couch. On auscultation, a scratching sound is heard — loudest over the lower left sternal edge, when the patient is

leaning forward. He also has a low-grade fever. He has a past medical history of a ST-elevation MI which was diagnosed, and treated with PCI, 6 weeks ago. What is the most likely diagnosis?

    A Viral pericarditis
    B Constrictive pericarditis
    C Cardiac tamponade
    D Dressler syndrome
    E Tietze syndrome

29. A 66-year old man has been experiencing pain in his right calf for the last 6 months. Initially, the pain would come about whenever he went for a walk, and it would be relieved by rest. However, over the last few weeks, he has experienced pain during rest. The pain is particularly bad at night, and he gets some relief from dangling his leg over the end of the bed. Recently, he has noticed a small, elliptical ulcer appear in between his toes on his right foot. He has a past medical history of ischaemic heart disease, and underwent a CABG 8 years ago. What is the most likely diagnosis?

    A Intermittent claudication
    B Critical limb ischaemia
    C Acute limb ischaemia
    D Leriche syndrome
    E Chronic deep vein thrombosis

30. A 3-year-old boy is brought, by his father, to see his GP because he has had a fever for the past 4 days and has cried in pain every time he has tried to eat. On examination, the patient's gums look red and swollen and there are small vesicles and ulcerations along the gumline. The GP suspects gingivostomatitis. What is the most likely cause?

    A Varicella
    B Primary HSV1 infection
    C Reactivation of HSV1
    D HSV2 infection
    E Infectious mononucleosis

Answers

1. A

To answer this question, you need a good understanding of the anatomy of the inguinal canal. It contains the spermatic cord in males and the round ligament in females. The inguinal ligament runs from the anterior superior iliac spine (ASIS) to the pubic tubercle, and forms the floor of the inguinal canal. The canal begins at the deep inguinal ring (located just above the midpoint of the inguinal ligament) and ends at the superficial inguinal ring (located just superior and medial to the pubic tubercle). Direct inguinal hernias arise from a weakness in the posterior wall of the inguinal canal, allowing abdominal viscera to protrude 'directly' through the back of the inguinal canal. In indirect inguinal hernias, the abdominal contents pass through the deep inguinal ring and along the inguinal canal. The hernial sacs in both conditions will protrude through the superficial ring and produce a swelling in the groin. These two types of hernia are differentiated on examination by reducing the hernia, placing a finger on the deep inguinal ring and asking the patient to cough. As you are blocking the deep inguinal ring with your finger, an indirect inguinal hernia should not reappear as a groin lump when the patient is asked to cough. Therefore, if the hernia appears again when the patient increases their intra-abdominal pressure (by coughing), it suggests that it is a direct inguinal hernia. This test is very crude and error prone — definitive diagnoses are often made in theatre.

Spigelian and obturator hernias are very rare. Spigelian hernias occur when abdominal contents herniate through the linea semilunaris, typically occurring inferior and lateral to the umbilicus. Obturator hernias occur through the obturator canal and they present with inner thigh pain when the hip is internally rotated (Howship–Romberg sign).

2. A

Aortic regurgitation normally causes an early diastolic murmur. However, severe aortic regurgitation leads to the regurgitated blood applying pressure on the mitral valve producing a low-pitched, rumbling mid-diastolic murmur, also known as an Austin-Flint murmur.

A Graham-Steell murmur is a high-pitched early diastolic murmur best heard at the upper left sternal edge. It is associated with pulmonary regurgitation. A Gibson murmur is a continuous 'machinery' murmur that is associated with patent ductus arteriosus. A Carey-Coombs murmur is a mid-diastolic murmur caused by turbulent blood flow over a thickened mitral valve. It is associated with acute rheumatic fever. A Barlow murmur is a mid-systolic click and an end-systolic murmur heard best at the apex and is associated with mitral valve prolapse.

3. D

Glasgow coma scale (GCS) criteria:

Eyes

1 — No eye opening
2 — Eyes open in response to pain
3 — Eyes open to verbal command
4 — Eyes open spontaneously

Verbal

1 — No verbal response
2 — Incomprehensible sounds
3 — Inappropriate responses
4 — Confused conversation
5 — Oriented

Motor

1 — No motor response
2 — Abnormal extension in response to pain (decerebrate posture)
3 — Abnormal flexion in response to pain (decorticate posture)
4 — Withdraws from pain
5 — Purposeful movement towards painful stimulus
6 — Obeys commands for movement

Minimum = 3; Maximum = 15

4. D

Minimal change disease is a type of non-proliferative glomerulonephritis which causes nephrotic syndrome in young children. Light microscopy shows no visible changes to the glomerulus (hence, minimal change), but electron microscopy shows diffuse loss of the processes of the podocytes in the Bowman's capsule. Membranous glomerulonephritis is another type of non-proliferative glomerulonephritis and is a cause of nephrotic syndrome in adults.

IgA nephropathy is the most common cause of glomerulonephritis and tends to occur a few days after upper respiratory tract infections. Henoch–Schönlein purpura is a type of IgA nephropathy that tends to affect older children and presents with a triad of abdominal pain, arthritis and a purpuric rash. IgA nephropathy and HSP cause nephritic syndrome — haematuria is more prominent than proteinuria. Rapidly progressive glomerulonephritis is an acute nephritic syndrome characterised by rapid loss of kidney function within weeks to months.

5. C

Myocardial infarctions in different areas of the heart produce different patterns of ST elevation on the ECG. Here is a list of the areas of the heart affected by an infarction along with the corresponding coronary artery and the ECG leads in which ST elevation will be observed.

Anterior MI — left anterior descending coronary artery — V1–4
Lateral MI — left circumflex coronary artery — aVL, I and V5–6
Inferior MI — right coronary artery — II, III and aVF
Posterior MI — posterior descending artery — ST depression in V1–4

6. C

Long-term pain and stiffness in both hands with swollen joints is an early presentation of rheumatoid arthritis (RA). RA is a chronic autoimmune inflammatory disease characterised by symmetrical polyarthritis, joint deformity and certain extra-articular manifestations (e.g. subcutaneous nodules, pulmonary fibrosis and episcleritis). Patients may also experience a degree of constitutional upset, such as weight loss, fatigue and a low-grade fever. On examination, tenderness and warmth of the metacarpophalangeal and proximal interphalangeal joints is often observed. The distal interphalangeal joints are spared. As the disease becomes more severe, the hands will become very deformed. Deformities that are typically seen in RA include radial deviation of the wrist, ulnar deviation of the fingers, Z deformity of the thumb swan neck deformity, Boutonnière deformity and trigger finger.

Reactive arthritis is a sterile arthritis that tends to occur days or weeks after a GI or urogenital infection. It presents with a triad of arthritis, uveitis and urethritis. Other extra-articular features of reactive arthritis include circinate balanitis and keratoderma blennorrhagicum. Osteoarthritis is a degenerative disease of the cartilage, usually occurring in weight-bearing joints such as the knees and hips. It is usually asymmetrical and the stiffness gets worse with activity. Psoriatic arthritis is the presence of arthritis in patients with psoriasis. There are five main forms of psoriatic arthritis (see Answers Section in Paper 4 for the 16th question).

7. C

Epigastric pain radiating to the back is suggestive of pancreatitis. The recurrent nature of this pain, weight loss and steatorrhoea (pale stools that are difficult to flush away) suggests that this is chronic pancreatitis. The steatorrhoea is caused by loss of exocrine function of the pancreas — lipases are unable to digest lipids in the small intestine so they move through the GI tract without being completely digested. It is important to remember that although acute pancreatitis is associated with very high serum amylase levels, chronic pancreatitis is typically associated with normal serum amylase. Faecal elastase is commonly used to investigate chronic pancreatitis — it is usually low in chronic pancreatitis, indicative of pancreatic exocrine insufficiency.

OGD is often used to investigate peptic ulcer disease, which is another common cause of epigastric pain. CA19-9 is the tumour marker for pancreatic cancer. Although it could be argued that the weight loss and epigastric discomfort could be caused by pancreatic cancer, this is less likely than chronic pancreatitis. Furthermore, SBAs about pancreatic cancer tend to mention the presence of painless jaundice and a palpable gallbladder (Courvoisier's Law). There are no signs of infection in this patient so blood cultures would be unnecessary.

8. B

The lung-related causes of shortness of breath (e.g. COPD, asthma, pneumonia) are often given plenty of attention but do not lose sight of the other, subtler, causes of shortness of breath. Anaemic patients have a reduced oxygen carrying capacity and, hence, they are more susceptible to hypoxia, which stimulates an increase in ventilatory drive. This patient is likely to be anaemic because of her heavy periods. This would cause gradual-onset shortness of breath as her anaemic blood struggles to supply her tissues with sufficient oxygen to meet demands. Hyperthyroidism leads to an increase in the metabolic rate of cells across the body, thereby increasing the oxygen demands of the body. This can result in an increase in ventilation in an attempt to keep up with these increased demands.

9. E

Hereditary haemochromatosis (HH) is an autosomal recessive disorder of iron metabolism caused by excessive intestinal absorption of dietary iron. This results in iron deposition in tissues and organs (e.g. skin, joints, liver, pancreas and adrenal glands). Iron is absorbed in the duodenum where it is either stored intracellularly bound to ferritin or transported out of the cells by ferroportin, a transmembrane protein. It then binds to transferrin in the blood stream. Hepcidin is a protein that inhibits ferroportin, thereby regulating the amount of iron entering the blood. 90% of cases of HH are caused by a mutation that leads to a deficiency of hepcidin, resulting in unregulated absorption of iron in the intestines. The main clinical features of HH are bronze skin, diabetes and hepatomegaly, due to iron deposition in the skin, pancreas and liver, respectively. It is investigated using iron studies — typical results in HH:

High Serum Iron — A deficiency of hepcidin leads to increased iron transport into the blood via ferroportin.

High Ferritin — Increased serum iron leads to an increase in ferritin in a compensatory attempt to increase intracellular iron storage.

Low Transferrin — Increased serum iron leads to decreased transferrin levels to prevent more iron from becoming plasma protein bound in the blood.

High Transferrin Saturation — Due to high serum iron and low transferrin.

Low Total Iron Binding Capacity (TIBC) — This is a measure of the blood's capacity to bind iron to transferrin. As transferrin is low, it is more difficult for iron to bind to transferrin.

N.B. The opposite changes in iron study results are observed in iron deficiency anaemia.

10. C

Osteoporosis is characterised by reduced bone mineral density (BMD) resulting in bone fragility and increased fracture risk. Osteoporosis can be a primary bone disorder of unknown cause. Secondary causes of osteoporosis include Cushing's syndrome, hyperthyroidism and hypogonadism. Post-menopausal women are at increased risk of osteoporosis due to the loss of the protective effect of oestrogen over bone. DEXA (dual energy X-ray absorptiometry) scans are the gold standard for diagnosing osteoporosis. It quantifies BMD based on the T-score (the number of standard deviations between the normal BMD for a young, healthy 30-year-old and the patient's BMD). T-scores are interpreted as follows:

$$0 \text{ to } -1 = \text{Normal}$$
$$-1 \text{ to } -2.5 = \text{Osteopaenia (at risk of developing into osteoporosis)}$$
$$-2.5 \text{ or worse} = \text{Osteoporosis}$$

11. D

The CHA_2DS_2-VASc score is used to assess the risk of stroke in patients with atrial fibrillation, and, hence, determine the benefit of long-term anticoagulation. It is based on the following factors:

Congestive heart failure

Hypertension

Age >75 yrs (2 points)

Diabetes mellitus

Stroke/TIA symptoms previously (2 points)

Vascular disease (e.g. peripheral artery disease)

Age 65–74 yrs (1 point)

Sex **c**ategory (Female = 1 point)

Guidelines recommend that patients with a score of 2 or more should be offered anticoagulation with warfarin or a DOAC (direct-acting oral anti-coagulant), previously known as NOACs (novel oral anticoagulants).

QRISK2 is used to predict the risk of cardiovascular disease based on traditional risk factors such as blood pressure and smoking status. It is used to decide whether to give primary prevention (e.g. statins). ABCD^2 predicts a patient's risk of stroke in the days following a TIA. This allows triaging of TIA patients and guides specialist referrals. GRACE score is used for risk assessment and triaging of patients with ACS. CURB-65 (Creatinine, Urea, Respiratory rate, Blood pressure, >65 yrs) is used to assess severity of community-acquired pneumonia. A score of 2 warrants hospital admission. A score of 3 or more is considered 'severe' pneumonia and should be considered for ITU admission.

12. B

Diabetic retinopathy is caused by progressive damage to blood vessels in the back of the eye. It occurs in a sequence: Background retinopathy → Pre-proliferative retinopathy → Proliferative retinopathy. A separate sub-type called maculopathy is when the disease affects the macula (an area in the centre of the retina responsible for central, high-resolution vision). Each of the types of diabetic retinopathy have distinctive features. Background retinopathy, the first in the continuum of diabetic retinopathy, features hard exudates (leaked lipid contents from blood vessels creating a cheesy yellow appearance), microaneurysms and blot haemorrhages. Pre-proliferative retinopathy is characterised by the presence of cotton wool spots — regions of retinal ischaemia. In proliferative retinopathy, new blood vessels begin to form in response to retinal ischaemia. If these vessels form near the macula, they can affect acuity and colour vision. Furthermore, they are fragile and prone to bleeding. In maculopathy, hard exudates are found near the macula. This can threaten direct vision.

13. D

Guillain–Barré syndrome (GBS) is an acute demyelinating polyneuro-pathy that often occurs a few weeks or months after an infection (e.g. *Campylobacter jejuni*). It results in ascending symmetrical muscle weakness. It is important to monitor forced vital capacity (FVC) using spirometry because GBS can cause respiratory muscle weakness, resulting in respiratory failure and, ultimately, death.

14. D

The British Thoracic Society has created a set of guidelines for the management of asthma, which are followed nationwide. Newly diagnosed asthma is first treated with a salbutamol (short-acting beta agonist) inhaler PRN (*'pro re nata'* — as and when it is needed). If the patient has to use the inhaler more than three times per week, they should see their GP in order to step up their management. With any asthma patient, it is important to ask about previous ITU admissions because this can help identify patients with particularly severe asthma. A simplified version of the BTS guidelines for asthma management are shown below:

STEP 1: Inhaled short-acting beta agonist (e.g. salbutamol)
STEP 2: Inhaled corticosteroid (e.g. beclomethasone)
STEP 3: Inhaled long-acting beta agonist (e.g. salmeterol) + consider increasing dose of inhaled corticosteroid
STEP 4: Consider trials of theophylline, oral beta agonists, oral leukotriene receptor antagonists (Montelukast therapy)
STEP 5: Oral corticosteroids

15. B

Causes of CKD include diabetes mellitus (most common), hypertension, idiopathic, glomerulonephritis, pyelonephritis, vasculitides, polycystic kidney disease, reflux nephropathy and obstructive nephropathy.

16. D

Polycythaemia refers to an abnormally high haemoglobin concentration. There are two main types — polycythaemia vera (a rare type of bone neoplasm resulting in a clonal proliferation of myeloid cells) and secondary polycythaemia (secondary to, for example, chronic hypoxia, renal tumours and erythropoietin abuse in athletes). The symptoms of polycythemia include headaches, tinnitus, blurred vision, history of thromboses, angina and, perhaps the most memorable symptom, pruritus after a hot bath.

Myelofibrosis is a disorder characterised by progressive bone marrow fibrosis, resulting in reduced bone marrow output, extramedullary haematopoiesis and massive splenomegaly. Myelofibrosis is often asymptomatic, however, there is a strong association between myelofibrosis and polycythaemia vera.

17. D

A young patient presenting acutely with right iliac fossa pain and vomiting is typical of appendicitis. Appendicitis is inflammation of the appendix that occurs following obstruction of the lumen of the appendix by a faecolith (calcified stone of faeces), foreign body, tumour, lymphoid hyperplasia or filarial worms. There are several signs of appendicitis that often come up in SBAs. The doctor in this question is eliciting psoas sign — achieved by lying the patient on their left-hand side, straightening their right leg and then passively extending their right hip. If pain is elicited, this suggests that the appendix is retrocaecal.

Rovsing's sign is when palpation of the left iliac fossa causes pain in the right iliac fossa. Obturator sign is pain on flexion and internal rotation of the hip and indicates that the appendix lies close to the obturator internus. Aaron's sign is referred as epigastric pain when pressure is applied over McBurney's point. Murphy's sign is the cessation of inspiration when two fingers are placed below the right costal margin in the midclavicular line and the patient is asked to take a deep breath in. This is suggestive of cholecystitis.

18. B

A squamous cell carcinoma (SCC) is one of the most common types of skin cancer. It is caused by malignant proliferation of keratinocytes. SCCs typically arise in sun-exposed areas and have raised, everted edges with an ulcerated centre and a keratotic core. A keratoacanthoma is a variant of SCC which grows rapidly but does not metastasise.

Basal cell carcinomas are the most common type of skin cancer. They have a classic description that is frequently seen in SBAs: A skin lesion with raised pearly edges and fine telangiectasia on the surface. It grows across the skin but never metastasises. Melanoma is the worst type of skin cancer and is often associated with a poor prognosis as it grows rapidly and metastasises early. It usually presents as an asymmetrical pigmented skin lesion with an irregular border. An actinic keratosis is a very common, non-malignant skin lesion that occurs due to sun damage. It has a thick, crusty surface.

19. D

Unruptured abdominal aortic aneurysms (AAA) are often asymptomatic and may be discovered incidentally. A normal aorta has a diameter of 2 cm. Aneurysms >5.5 cm in diameter are more likely to rupture, so surgery, either by open repair or endovascular aneurysm repair (EVAR), is usually recommended. EVAR has a lower morbidity and mortality but a higher rate of graft complications, therefore, it is usually used in elderly patients. NHS Choices recommends regular surveillance for patients with an AAA diameter of 3–4.5 cm (every year) and 4.5–5.4 cm (every 3 months). Despite these guidelines, patients are often reviewed at MDT and treated on an individualised basis.

20. C

Diabetes insipidus (DI) results in the production of large volumes of dilute urine and is caused by insufficient production of vasopressin (central DI) or the inability of the kidneys to respond to vasopressin (nephrogenic DI). DI is investigated using a water deprivation test during which the patient is not allowed to drink water for 8 hrs whilst urine osmolality is measured every 2 hrs and weight is monitored every 1 hr. An increase in urine osmolality (>600 mOsm/kg) is a normal physiological response to dehydration — this will be seen in patients with psychogenic polydipsia, as this is not caused by endocrine dysfunction. Failure to concentrate urine with water deprivation indicates DI. When desmopressin (vasopressin analogue) is administered, it would cause an increase in urine osmolality in patients with central DI (because their kidneys are still responsive to desmopressin), however, it would cause little or no change in patients with nephrogenic DI.

21. C

Kaposi's sarcoma is a systemic disease caused by infection with human herpesvirus 8 (HHV-8), presenting as cutaneous tumours. It is an AIDS-defining illness that is often the first AIDS-related complication in HIV patients. Lesions appear mainly on the extremities, but can occur on the trunk, back, face and mucous membranes. Organ involvement is sometimes present in the gastrointestinal and respiratory tract and can result in death. Other important AIDS-defining illnesses include candidiasis (of the oesophagus, trachea, bronchi or lungs), cervical cancer, Burkitt's lymphoma, cytomegalovirus retinitis, mycobacterium avium complex, *Pneumocystis jiroveci* pneumonia and toxoplasmosis.

22. A

Paracetamol overdose, although initially asymptomatic, can cause extensive hepatic necrosis and requires urgent treatment. Paracetamol levels are measured 4 hrs post-ingestion, the result is then plotted on a graph and if the paracetamol level is above a certain level, IV n-acetylcysteine is administered.

Other overdoses and antidotes:

> Opiate Overdose — Naloxone
> Benzodiazepine Overdose — Flumezanil
> Organophosphate Poisoning — Atropine
> Aspirin Overdose — Sodium Bicarbonate

23. B

Haemolytic uraemic syndrome (HUS) is a triad of microangiopathic haemolytic anaemia (MAHA), acute renal failure and thrombocytopaenia. It most often occurs following a diarrhoeal infection by *E. coli* O157 in children. In simple terms, HUS results from endothelial injury leading to activation of platelets and the clotting cascade, which, in turn, leads to small-vessel thrombosis. Glomeruli are particularly vulnerable, hence why HUS leads to acute renal failure. The small vessel thromboses also cause intravascular haemolysis by exerting shear forces on the blood cells. This patient has a recent history of diarrhoeal illness with a stool culture identifying *E. coli* O157, schistocytes (red cell fragments) indicating intravascular haemolysis and a significant rise in creatinine, indicating acute renal failure.

N.B. The clotting screen is normal in HUS.

Although MAHA is a component of HUS, it is not the best answer in this case because this patient has other features that are typical of HUS. Thrombotic thrombocytopaenic purpura (TTP) has the same features as HUS with the addition of fever and fluctuating neurological signs. Disseminated intravascular coagulation (DIC) is widespread activation of the clotting cascade resulting in low platelets, low Hb and low fibrinogen with a high APTT/PT.

24. B

Atypical pneumonia, to put it simply, is a type of pneumonia that is not caused by the 'typical' pathogens and does not present like a 'typical' pneumonia. It tends to present with vague symptoms such as malaise, headache and diarrhoea. The three main causes of atypical pneumonia are *Legionella pneumophila*, *Mycoplasma pneumoniae* and *Chlamydia psittaci*. These present with the vague symptoms listed above, however, they each have a distinguishing feature. *L. pneumophila* is found in bodies of water kept at temperatures below 60°C, such as air conditioning units, and it is associated with causing confusion. *L. pneumophila* also produces antigens that are excreted in the patient's urine. Since this patient has recently returned from a business trip, it is possible that he was exposed to *Legionella* via a contaminated air conditioning unit in a hotel. Therefore, the best investigation would be to test for urinary antigens. *Mycoplasma pneumoniae* causes red cell agglutination and is associated with transverse myelitis. *Chlamydia psittaci* is primarily found in birds but can cause an atypical pneumonia, known as 'Psittacosis', in humans that are exposed to birds.

25. B

Most cancers are staged using the TNM classification, however, some cancers have specific staging systems. Gleason staging helps evaluate the prognosis of patients with prostate cancer based on the histological appearance of a prostate biopsy.

Breslow thickness is a prognostic indicator for melanoma based on the depth to which tumour cells have invaded surrounding tissues. The GRACE score is used to risk stratify patients who have suffered an acute coronary syndrome. The Wells score allows assessment of pre-test probability in patients with a suspected pulmonary embolism. Dukes' staging is used for colorectal cancer.

26. A

In symptomatic UTI patients with positive nitrites or leukocytes on urinalysis, empirical antibiotic treatment should be commenced whilst awaiting the sensitivities from an MSU. In non-pregnant women with uncomplicated UTI (normal urinary tract structure and function), trimethoprim or nitrofurantoin are commonly used. Alternative treatment options include co-amoxiclav or cephalexin. Pregnant women with UTIs require specialist attention because conventional treatment options (e.g. trimethoprim, a folate antagonist) may cause harm to a foetus. Men have a much longer urethra so have a lower risk of getting a UTI. Therefore, UTIs in men should be taken seriously as it often results from some form of anomaly. Men with symptoms of an upper UTI, recurrent UTIs or failure to respond to treatment should be referred to an urologist.

27. E

All available options may present with PR bleeding and pruritus ani — however, they can be distinguished based on the examination findings. A lump that protrudes with defecation and requires manual reduction suggests haemorrhoids or rectal prolapse. Grades of haemorrhoids:

Grade 1: no prolapse
Grade 2: prolapse on defecation but reduces spontaneously
Grade 3: prolapse requires manual reduction
Grade 4: remain persistently prolapsed and cannot be reduced

As the prolapse can be reduced manually after defecation, at this point, grade 3 haemorrhoids and rectal prolapse are the top differentials. Type 1 rectal prolapse occurs when only the rectal mucosa protrudes through the anus and type 2 occurs when all layers of the rectum protrude through the anus, creating a mass which has palpable, concentric muscular rings. Some patients report constipation, but fecal incontinence is more common due to the lax anal tone. Some also report a mucus discharge. The two main causes of rectal prolapse are lax anal tone (usually due to pudendal nerve damage) and prolonged straining. The lax anal tone and palpation of muscular rings on examination makes this most likely to be a type 2 rectal prolapse.

28. D

Dressler's syndrome is a type of pericarditis that arises 2–10 weeks after an MI. It is thought that injury to the myocardium during an MI stimulates the production of autoantibodies against heart muscle. These autoantibodies cause pericardial inflammation many weeks later. It presents in the same way as viral pericarditis — pleuritic chest pain that is relieved by sitting forward, fever and a pericardial rub. Dressler's should not be confused with a simple post-MI pericarditis which occurs within 2–4 days of an MI. Dressler's is treated with analgesia and anti-inflammatories (e.g. NSAIDs). It may cause a pericardial effusion, which may require pericardiocentesis.

29. B

Peripheral vascular disease (PVD) is an umbrella term used to describe the diseases that result from progressive stenosis of peripheral arteries due to atherosclerosis. Intermittent claudication is a cramping pain in the lower limb muscles that occurs on exercise and is relieved by rest. Critical limb ischaemia is a more severe form of PVD characterised by rest pain, night pain and tissue loss (e.g. arterial ulcers, gangrene). This patient has all the main features of critical limb ischaemia. Leriche syndrome is a type of intermittent claudication resulting in buttock claudication, erectile dysfunction and weak distal pulses, due to aortoiliac stenosis. Patients with PVD usually have a history of atherosclerotic disease (e.g. ischaemic heart disease). PVD can be diagnosed using ABPI: 0.5–0.9 = peripheral vascular disease; <0.5 = critical limb ischaemia.

Acute limb ischaemia is caused by sudden cessation of blood flow to a limb by a thrombus or embolus (usually from AF). Chronic DVT causes leg swelling, pain and skin discolouration.

30. B

Herpes simplex virus (HSV) is a dsDNA virus that is transmitted via close contact with an individual shedding the virus in oral secretions. Most HSV1 infections are acquired during early childhood and the infection is lifelong. Primary infection is mostly asymptomatic, but may cause pharyngitis, gingivostomatitis and herpetic whitlow (digital blisters/pustules). Following primary infection, HSV1 becomes dormant, classically in the trigeminal ganglia. Reactivation may occur due to physical or emotional stress or immunosuppression, and presents as herpes labialis (cold sores). HSV2 is almost exclusively sexually transmitted and it causes genital herpes (presenting with genital or anal blisters, often with dysuria, fever and malaise). Varicella (chickenpox) is a primary infection with varicella zoster virus. It causes an intensely itchy and spreading rash affecting mainly the face and trunk. Infectious mononucleosis (glandular fever) is an infection caused by Epstein–Barr virus, presenting with sore throat, fever, lymphadenopathy, tonsillar enlargement and splenomegaly.

Paper 2

Questions

1. A 31-year-old man presents to his GP with a 2-day history of central chest pain, which gets worse when he breathes in and when exercising. Cardiovascular and respiratory examinations detect no abnormalities, however, the patient winces in pain when the GP palpates for heaves and thrills. What is the most likely diagnosis?

   A Pulmonary embolism
   B Myocarditis
   C Tension pneumothorax
   D Costochondritis
   E Pleurisy

2. Which of the following is unlikely to cause pleuritic chest pain?

   A Tension pneumothorax
   B Rib fracture
   C Pulmonary fibrosis
   D Pneumonia
   E Pericarditis

3. A 28-year-old PhD student books an appointment to see her GP about some small lumps on her groin. On closer inspection, there are

multiple small, firm, dome-shaped lumps with an umbilicated centre. On direct questioning, she reveals that she has recently had a new sexual partner. What is the most likely diagnosis?

    A Molluscum contagiosum
    B Varicella zoster
    C Syphilis
    D Gonorrhoea
    E Sebaceous cysts

4. A 71-year-old woman presents to A&E with a headache that has gradually been getting worse over the past week. The pain is localised over the left half of her forehead and does not radiate. She has also been eating less frequently as her jaw becomes painful when she chews her food. On direct questioning, she admits to experiencing some stiffness and pain in her shoulders over the past 6 months. On examination, she has a thickened, non-pulsatile temporal artery. What is the first step in her management?

    A Check ESR
    B Temporal artery biopsy
    C IV hydrocortisone
    D Oral prednisolone
    E IV antibiotics

5. A 24-year-old female, who has recently returned from a 3-week trip to Vietnam, complains that she has been feeling 'under the weather' with fevers and joint pain. On direct questioning, she reveals that she had unprotected sexual intercourse with a stranger whilst in Vietnam. She is jaundiced and has right upper quadrant tenderness. Hepatitis B serology is requested. The results are shown below:

    HBsAg+
    HBeAg−
    HBcAb IgM+
    HBcAb IgG+
    HBsAb−

What is the hepatitis status of this patient?

    A Acute infection
    B Chronic infection
    C Cleared
    D Vaccinated
    E Susceptible

6. An 18-year-old female is brought to A&E, by ambulance, having been involved in a road traffic accident. She has bled significantly and needs an urgent blood transfusion. Her blood group is AB+. Which of the following blood groups will she be able to accept?

    A A+
    B AB−
    C B−
    D O−
    E All of the above

7. Which clinical test can be used to diagnose ankylosing spondylitis?

    A Schober's test
    B Schirmir's test
    C Buerger's test
    D Weber's test
    E Tensilon test

8. A 53-year-old Afro-Caribbean man visits the GP to have his blood pressure measured. He has a history of hypertension and has been taking Amlodipine for 6 months. His blood pressure is 162/110 mm Hg. The GP is not satisfied with his blood pressure control and wants to step up his management. Which medication should be added?

    A Verapamil
    B Spironolactone
    C Bendroflumethiazide
    D Doxazosin
    E Enalapril

9. An 81-year-old man has been urinating about 12 times every day, including at night, and has difficulty starting a stream, which he describes as being 'very weak'. He has also suffered from lower back pain over the past month. A DRE is performed, revealing an asymmetrically enlarged, nodular prostate gland. Which investigation is most likely to provide a definitive diagnosis?

   A PSA
   B Acid phosphatase
   C Transrectal ultrasound-guided biopsy
   D CT scan
   E Isotope bone scan

10. A 61-year-old man is brought to A&E by his daughter as he has become increasingly breathless over the past 24 hrs and he has been coughing up a large amount of green sputum. He has a past medical history of COPD. Arterial blood gases are requested which show the following results (on room air):

    pH: 7.33 (7.35–7.45)
    PaO_2: 6.7 kPa (> 10.6 kPa on air)
    $PaCO_2$: 9.6 kPa (4.7–6 kPa on air)
    HCO_3^-: 33 mmol/L (22–28 mmol/L)
    Respiratory Rate: 22/min

    What is the diagnosis?

    A Partially compensated respiratory acidosis
    B Fully compensated respiratory acidosis
    C Partially compensated metabolic acidosis
    D Fully compensated metabolic acidosis
    E Acute type 1 respiratory failure

11. A 73-year-old man has come to the outpatient clinic with his wife. She says that her husband seems very confused on some days and then seems completely normal on others. During the consultation, the

patient appears confused with an AMTS of 4/10. He is distressed and claims that he can see little men running across the desk towards him. The doctor also notices a resting tremor. What is the most likely diagnosis?

    A Lewy body dementia
    B Alzheimer's disease
    C Depressive pseudodementia
    D Frontotemporal dementia
    E Vascular dementia

12. A 47-year-old man has gained 10 kg of weight over the past 2 months, and he has also been feeling more depressed and irritable than usual. On examination, he has a round face and striae across his abdomen. Following investigation, a diagnosis of Cushing's syndrome is made. Which test can help distinguish between Cushing's disease and other causes of Cushing's syndrome (e.g. ectopic ACTH)?

    A 24-hr urinary free cortisol
    B Random plasma cortisol
    C Low-dose dexamethasone suppression test
    D High-dose dexamethasone suppression test
    E Midnight cortisol

13. The red reflex is an important part of the ophthalmological examination. Which of the following conditions can result in loss of the red reflex?

    A Herpes simplex keratitis
    B Cataract
    C Astigmatism
    D Conjunctivitis
    E Aniridia

14. A 32-year-old man presents to his GP with an 8-month history of diffuse abdominal pain and frequent loose motions. He has also been

passing blood with his stools. On examination, a red ring around the cornea is seen in both eyes. The patient is referred for a colonoscopy and biopsy. What would you expect the biopsy to show?

    A Non-caseating granulomas
    B Eosinophilic infiltration
    C Villous atrophy and crypt hyperplasia
    D High-grade dysplasia and metaplastic columnar epithelium
    E Mucosal ulcers, goblet cell depletion and crypt abscesses

15. A 28-year-old professional cyclist visits his GP complaining of headaches and blurred vision. He is worried that his symptoms will affect his performance in an important race in 3 weeks' time. On direct questioning, he admits to taking 'performance enhancers' in preparation for his race. On examination, scratch marks are seen on his trunk. What is the most likely diagnosis?

    A Thalassaemia
    B Polycythaemia rubra vera
    C Secondary polycythaemia
    D Hodgkin's lymphoma
    E Non-Hodgkin's lymphoma

16. A 22-year-old teacher visits her GP after fainting several times over the past 2 months. She does not experience any palpitations, lightheadedness or auras before she faints, and she recovers very quickly. She has not bitten her tongue or become incontinent at any point. When questioned about the timing of these episodes, she reveals that she has only ever collapsed at work after she has been writing on the whiteboard for quite some time. On examination, a firm, immobile lump is palpated in her left supraclavicular fossa. What is the most likely diagnosis?

    A Paroxysmal atrial fibrillation
    B Transient ischaemic attack
    C Atonic seizures
    D Subclavian steal syndrome
    E Vasovagal syncope

17. Which of the following triads best describes the main features of nephrotic syndrome?

    A Proteinuria, Hypoalbuminaemia, Oedema
    B Haematuria, Hypoalbuminaemia, Oedema
    C Proteinuria, Haematuria, Hyperlipidaemia
    D Proteinuria, Haematuria, Hypoalbuminaemia
    E Frequency, Urgency, Dysuria

18. A 63-year-old man with ascending bilateral limb weakness and ascending paraesthesia is diagnosed with Guillain–Barré syndrome. Three weeks prior to the onset of these symptoms, he suffered from gastroenteritis. Which organism is most likely to have caused this infection?

    A *Salmonella*
    B *Campylobacter jejuni*
    C *E. coli* O157
    D Rotavirus
    E *Entamoeba histolytica*

19. A 79-year-old care home resident is admitted to hospital with a 4-day history of a cough productive of green sputum. She has also experienced some chest pain and shortness of breath. A chest X-ray shows an area of consolidation in the right middle lobe with a right-sided pleural effusion. What is the most appropriate treatment option?

    A Co-amoxiclav and clarithromycin
    B Co-trimoxazole
    C Metronidazole
    D Flucloxacillin
    E Rifampicin and isoniazid

20. A 76-year-old care home resident has fractured his neck of femur having fallen out of bed. He is referred to the orthopaedic surgery department and undergoes an operation. Post-operatively, he is in

considerable pain and is given 5 mg morphine sulphate. Which of these side-effects is he most likely to experience?

    A Constipation
    B Blurred vision
    C Cough
    D Tremor
    E Rash

21. A 65-year-old man, who is currently undergoing treatment for chronic lymphocytic leukaemia, presents with an extremely painful left great toe. On closer inspection, he has a fiercely inflamed left metatarsophalangeal joint. He has no other symptoms. What would you expect to see on analysis of the joint fluid aspirate?

    A High WCC, turbid fluid
    B Positively birefringent, rhomboid-shaped crystals
    C Positively birefringent, needle-shaped crystals
    D Negatively birefringent, rhomboid-shaped crystals
    E Negatively birefringent, needle-shaped crystals

22. A 47-year-old woman has had several 'dizzy spells' over the past 6 weeks. She has been feeling very faint when getting out of bed in the morning and has also experienced some vague abdominal pain along with weight loss and lethargy. Examination reveals dark palmar creases and vitiligo on her back. What is the most appropriate investigation to request?

    A Full blood count
    B Fasting blood glucose
    C ECG
    D Short synacthen test
    E Thyroid function test

23. A 78-year-old woman visits her GP with a 4-month history of constipation and blood coating her stools. She has also lost 9 kg of weight

and complains that she doesn't 'feel empty' after defecating. Abdominal examination is normal, apart from an enlarged left supra-clavicular lymph node. What is the most likely diagnosis?

    A Cancer of the rectum
    B Cancer of the sigmoid colon
    C Gastric carcinoma
    D Cancer of the caecum
    E Pancreatic cancer

24. A 75-year-old man is rushed into A&E by ambulance. He finds it difficult to answer simple questions and is struggling to speak. On examination, power is 2/5 in his right arm, 4/5 in his right leg and 5/5 in his left arm and leg. He has marked facial muscle weakness on the right half of his face and he is blind in the right half of his visual field. A CT head scan is performed and an ischaemic stroke is diagnosed. Which artery is most likely to be involved?

    A Right anterior cerebral artery
    B Left anterior cerebral artery
    C Right posterior cerebral artery
    D Right middle cerebral artery
    E Left middle cerebral artery

25. A 62-year-old diabetic on metformin sees his GP for a routine blood test. He claims that he has been compliant with his treatment and has not experienced any symptoms recently. His blood test reveals:

    Na^+: 116 mmol/L (135–145)
    K+: 3.7 mmol/L (3.5–5)
    Ca^{2+}: 2.4 mmol/L (2.2–2.6)
    Total Cholesterol: 9.2 mmol/L (<5)
    Serum Albumin: 48 g/L (35–50)
    TFT — Normal
    SST — Normal

What is the most likely cause of his hyponatraemia?

    A Addison's disease
    B Hypothyroidism
    C Pseudohyponatraemia
    D Drug side-effect
    E Nephrotic syndrome

26. Which of the following lung pathologies produces the 'sail sign' appearance on CXR?

    A Right upper lobe collapse
    B Right middle lobe collapse
    C Right lower lobe collapse
    D Left upper lobe collapse
    E Left lower lobe collapse

27. A 47-year-old man has vomited three times and has not passed any faeces or flatus for the last 4 days. He had an open cholecystectomy 6 years ago but has otherwise been relatively fit and healthy. What is the best immediate management option for this patient?

    A NG tube and IV fluids
    B Surgery to resolve the obstruction
    C Gastrograffin
    D IV antibiotics
    E Reassure and discharge

28. A 24-year-old man has been invited for a follow-up appointment with his GP after his blood pressure was elevated on two previous occasions. When his blood pressure is measured again, it reads 178/96 mm Hg. Before discussing management options, the GP performs a cardiovascular examination. No abnormalities were

detected except for a radio-femoral delay. What is the most likely diagnosis?

    A Conn's syndrome
    B Renal artery stenosis
    C Aortic dissection
    D Aortic transection
    E Coarctation of the aorta

29. A 46-year-old female has experienced a painful sensation on the outer side of her left thigh for the past 3 months. She mentions that the sensation is very 'bizarre' and sometimes feels like it is burning or tingling. She has no other symptoms and has no past medical history of note. What is the most likely diagnosis?

    A Meralgia paraesthetica
    B Multiple sclerosis
    C Sciatica
    D Peripheral neuropathy
    E Disc herniation

30. A 47-year-old female suffering from RUQ pain, lethargy and pruritus, is found to have an ALP of 300 IU/L (30–150 IU/L) and serology is positive for anti-mitochondrial antibodies. She also complains of dry, itchy eyes. Examination findings include icterus and xanthelasma. What is the most likely diagnosis?

    A Type 1 autoimmune hepatitis
    B Type 2 autoimmune hepatitis
    C Primary sclerosing cholangitis
    D Primary biliary cirrhosis
    E Cirrhosis

Answers

1. D

Costochondritis is acute inflammation of the costal cartilage. It is usually idiopathic. Tietze's syndrome is a form of costochondritis characterised by painful swelling of the costal cartilage. Costochondritis usually presents with chest pain and tenderness on palpation either side of the sternum. The pain often gets worse when coughing, on deep inspiration or during exercise. PE, tension pneumothorax, myocarditis and pleurisy will also cause pleuritic pain, however, it is likely that other abnormalities will also be identified on cardiovascular and respiratory examination.

2. C

Pleuritic chest pain is described as 'a sharp, stabbing pain that gets worse when breathing in or coughing'. The causes of pleuritic chest pain are remembered as the **5 Ps**: **P**E, **p**neumothorax, **p**ericarditis, **p**leurisy and **p**neumonia. Other causes of pleuritic chest pain include subphrenic pathology (e.g. abscess), rib fractures and costochondritis.

3. A

Molluscum contagiosum is a skin condition caused by a pox virus. It mainly occurs in children and is spread via skin-to-skin contact. In adults, it tends to be transmitted via sexual contact and occurs on the lower abdomen and genital area. The skin lesions are typically described as dome-shaped, firm and smooth with an umbilicated centre. The lesions will last for around 8 months.

Varicella zoster virus (VZV) causes chicken pox (in children) and shingles (in adults). Chicken pox is characterised by the sudden appearance of an extremely itchy rash. The vesicles appear, weep and crust over. It is also often accompanied by prodromal flu-like symptoms. Shingles is caused by reactivation of VZV (during times of stress), which lies dormant in dorsal root ganglia after primary infection. It causes tingling and painful skin lesions in a dermatomal distribution. Syphilis is a sexually-transmitted disease caused by *Treponema pallidum*. It begins as a single painless genital ulcer, which is followed by generalised lymphadenopathy and widespread skin lesions. Tertiary syphilis is when the infection spreads to the brain and causes neurological complications. Gonorrhoea is another sexually-transmitted infection, caused by *Neisseria gonorrhoeae*, which presents with vaginal or urethral discharge, dysuria and dyspareunia (in women). A sebaceous cyst is a keratinous, epithelium-lined cyst arising from a blocked hair follicle. They are very common and appear as smooth lumps with an overlying punctum that may discharge a creamy substance.

4. A

Temporal arteritis (also known as giant cell arteritis) is a large-vessel vasculitis that typically presents with a unilateral headache, scalp tenderness and jaw claudication. There may also be systemic features such as malaise, fever and weight loss. Temporal arteritis, if left untreated, can cause irreversible loss of vision (due to ophthalmic artery involvement) so it must be treated urgently with oral prednisolone. However, as the side-effects of high-dose steroids are not warranted in patients who do not actually have temporal arteritis, checking ESR is advised as the first step in the management. Although ESR is not specific to temporal arteritis, it is highly unlikely that a patient with a normal ESR has temporal arteritis. In addition, the ESR result can be turned around rapidly so the consequences of delaying treatment to measure ESR are relatively minor. If the ESR is raised, the patient should be given high-dose oral prednisolone. A temporal artery biopsy showing inflammatory changes is diagnostic of temporal arteritis. However, there is a risk of false-negatives because the biopsy may not sample the affected tissue. The biopsy result can take a long time to process, so this should not delay treatment.

5. A

Hepatitis B serology is often poorly understood by many medical students. Hepatitis B virus (HBV) is prevalent in sub-Saharan Africa and Southeast Asia. It is transmitted via sexual contact, blood (e.g. contaminated needles) and vertical transmission from mother to child. To understand hepatitis serology, it is important to appreciate the location of the antigens. HBV is a small DNA virus composed of an outer envelope which contains surface antigen (HBsAg). This surrounds a nucleocapsid that encloses the viral DNA. The nucleocapsid carries the core antigen (HBcAg) which is involved in viral replication. The e antigen (HbeAg) is also closely associated with the nucleocapsid.

HBsAg is administered in the hepatitis B vaccine. The immune system will generate antibodies against the surface antigen — HBsAb. HBsAg will eventually be cleared from the system but HBsAb will persist. Therefore, individuals that have been vaccinated against hepatitis B will only be HBsAb+. Previously infected patients who have cleared the virus will be HBsAb+ and HBcAb IgG+.

The earliest mark of acute infection will be a rise in HBsAg. This will be followed by a rise in HbcAb IgM and HBcAb IgG. HBcAb IgM will only be present during the acute phase of the infection. HBcAb IgG will persist once the virus is cleared or if the infection becomes chronic. HBeAg can be present in both acute and chronic infection — it tends to be used as a marker of infectivity and to monitor response to treatment. In summary, acute infection will cause HBsAg+, HBsAb−, HBcAb IgM+, HBcAb IgG+ and HBeAg +/−.

If HBsAg is detected in the serum 6 months after an acute infection, it suggests that the patient has developed chronic hepatitis B. These patients will also have HBcAb IgG and may have HBeAg. In summary, chronic infection will cause HBsAg+, HBsAb−, HBcAb IgM−, HBcAb IgG+ and HBeAg +/−. Finally, susceptible individuals will be negative in all components of hepatitis B serology.

As the patient is HBsAg+, he has either an acute or chronic infection. The presence of HBcAb IgM means that this is an acute infection. A table summarising hepatitis B serology is shown below:

	HBsAg	HBeAg	HBcAb IgM	HBcAb IgG	HBsAb
Susceptible	−	−	−	−	−
Acute	+	+/−	+	+	−
Chronic	+	+/−	−	+	−
Cleared	−	−	−	+	+
Vaccinated	−	−	−	−	+

6. E

There are four main blood types, defined by the ABO system. As a general principle, the immune system will generate antibodies against the red blood cell antigens that are not present on the host red blood cells.

> Group A has A antigens, produces anti-B antibodies
>
> Group B has B antigens, produces anti-A antibodies
>
> Group AB has A & B antigens, produces no antibodies against A or B antigens
>
> Group O has no antigens, produces anti-A and anti-B antibodies

Red cells may also have Rhesus (RhD) antigen. If present, your blood type is described as Rhesus 'positive'. This patient is AB+ meaning that she has A, B and RhD antigens. Therefore, she has no antibodies against the main red cell antigens, and, hence, can accept blood of any type without causing a transfusion reaction. Conversely, O− patients have antibodies against A, B and RhD antigens, so they can only accept O− blood. As everyone can accept O− blood, they are referred to as 'universal donors'.

7. A

Ankylosing spondylitis is a seronegative spondyloarthropathy that presents with lower back pain and stiffness that is worst in the morning and improves with activity. It leads to a reduced range of spinal motion, which can be detected using Schober's test. During this clinical test, a mark is made on the skin overlying the fifth lumbar spinous process (usually at the level of the posterior superior iliac spine) and a second mark is made 10 cm above the first. The patient is then asked to bend over, which flexes the spine. In normal subjects, the distance between the two marks will increase to >15 cm. If the distance is less than 15 cm, this indicates a reduction in spinal flexion, which supports a diagnosis of ankylosing spondylitis.

Schirmer's test assesses tear production in patients with Sjögren's syndrome. Buerger's test is used to demonstrate peripheral vascular disease. Weber's test, when used in combination with Rinne's test, can differentiate between conductive and sensorineural hearing loss. The Tensilon test involves administering a very short-acting acetylcholinesterase inhibitor to diagnose myasthenia gravis by demonstrating by a rapid improvement in muscle weakness.

8. E

NICE defines hypertension as a blood pressure consistently >140/90 mm Hg. If this is found during ambulatory blood pressure monitoring (ABPM), patients should be considered for treatment. Learn the management guidelines for hypertension as it commonly comes up in SBAs and OSCEs.

Lifestyle interventions should be encouraged and includes maintaining a healthy diet with reduced sodium intake, regular exercise, reducing caffeine and alcohol consumption and stopping smoking. The NICE guidelines for treating hypertension are simplified below:

STEP 1: Patients <55 years old should be offered an ACE inhibitor (ACEI e.g. enalapril) or angiotensin receptor blocker (ARB e.g. losartan). Patients >55 years old and patients of Afro-Caribbean origin should be offered a calcium channel blocker (CCB e.g. amlodipine) or, if there is any evidence (or high risk) of heart failure, a thiazide-like diuretic (e.g. bendroflumethiazide).

STEP 2: Offer a CCB with an ACEI or ARB. If CCBs are not suitable, a thiazide-like diuretic can be used instead.

STEP 3: Offer a combination of an ACEI or ARB with a CCB and a thiazide-like diuretic.

STEP 4: If these three steps are unsuccessful in gaining control of blood pressure, it is considered 'resistant hypertension'. Expert help should be sought and a fourth antihypertensive may be added e.g. spironolactone.

NICE guidelines aim for an average blood pressure below 135/85 mm Hg for people under the age of 80 and below 145/85 mm Hg for people over the age of 80.

9. C

Diseases of the prostate gland typically present with lower urinary tract symptoms (LUTS), which can be divided into storage and voiding symptoms. These can be remembered using the mnemonic **FUN** (storage) **WISE** (voiding): Frequency, Urgency, Nocturia, Weak stream, Intermittency, Straining, incomplete Emptying. Other features include terminal dribbling, urinary retention and overflow incontinence. Prostate cancer can also cause symptoms due to metastasis (e.g. back pain due to bone metastases), paraneoplastic syndromes (e.g. hypercalcaemia) and constitutional upset (e.g. weight loss, malaise). Transrectal ultrasound (TRUS) guided biopsy allows a histological analysis of the prostate tissue, which can most reliably confirm a diagnosis of prostate cancer.

Prostate-specific antigen (PSA) is used as a screening test for prostate cancer, however, it is not very specific. Acid phosphatase was used as a screening test for prostate cancer before the introduction of PSA. A CT scan may be useful, once the diagnosis is confirmed, to assess the extent of local invasion and lymph node involvement. An isotope bone scan may be used to check for bone metastases.

10. A

Arterial blood gases (ABG) can be confusing at first but they are very quick to analyse once you learn the step-by-step approach to ABGs.

1) What is the pH? Is it an acidosis or an alkalosis?
2) What is the $PaCO_2$? *Note*: CO_2 is acidic
   a. High + Acidosis = respiratory acidosis
   b. Low + Acidosis = metabolic acidosis (low CO_2 is attempting to compensate)
   c. High + Alkalosis = metabolic alkalosis (high CO_2 is attempting to compensate)
   d. Low + Alkalosis = respiratory alkalosis
3) What is the HCO_3^-? *Note*: HCO_3^- is alkaline
   a. High + Alkalosis = metabolic alkalosis

   b. Low + Alkalosis = respiratory alkalosis (low HCO_3^- is
      attempting to compensate)

   c. High + Acidosis = respiratory acidosis (high HCO_3^- is
      attempting to compensate)

   d. Low + Acidosis = metabolic acidosis

   e. HCO_3^- may be low in acute acidosis as it acts as a buffer by
      sequestering the excess H+ ions

N.B. Other metabolic acids (e.g. lactic acid, ketoacids) are difficult to measure directly but can cause a metabolic acidosis, when in excess. The 'anion gap', seen in most ABG results, is an indirect estimate of the levels of these metabolic acids. If the anion gap is high, it suggests that one of these metabolic acids is in excess, and, therefore, is causing the metabolic acidosis.

11. A

To summarise the clinical picture, this patient is experiencing fluctuating levels of confusion, hallucinations and a resting tremor. These are the major features of Lewy body dementia (also known as dementia with Lewy bodies (DLB)). Hallucinations are the distinguishing feature, commonly mentioned in SBAs. DLB is characterised by the accumulation of abnormal aggregates of proteins, called Lewy bodies in the cytoplasm of neurons. It also leads to a loss of dopaminergic neurons in the substantia nigra, resulting in features of parkinsonism (resting tremor, postural instability, bradykinesia and rigidity). DLB is the second most common form of dementia behind Alzheimer's disease, which causes the typical dementia symptoms, such as anterograde amnesia, confusion, changes in personality and mood and difficulty planning. Frontotemporal dementia tends to first present with a change in personality or behaviour. Vascular dementia is caused by multiple small cerebral infarcts, leading to a loss of brain function. Patients may have a history of experiencing stroke-like symptoms. The patient's state tends to undergo a stepwise decline in vascular dementia. Depressive pseudodementia is when dementia-like symptoms result from underlying depression. SBAs are likely to mention a recent bereavement or traumatic life event when alluding to depressive pseudodementia.

12. D

When a patient initially presents with symptoms suggestive of Cushing's syndrome, it is important to first confirm the diagnosis of Cushing's syndrome before searching for a cause. This can be done using a variety of tests such as 24-hr urinary free cortisol, midnight cortisol, and a low-dose dexamethasone suppression test. The 24-hr urinary free cortisol and midnight cortisol are often inaccurate due to measurement issues, variations in the patient's circadian rhythm and stress levels. The low-dose dexamethasone suppression test involves administering dexamethasone 0.5 mg/6 hrs PO for 2 days — serum cortisol is measured at 0 and 48 hrs and a lack of suppression (<50 nmol/L) is observed in Cushing's syndrome. A high-dose dexamethasone suppression test involves administering dexamethasone 2 mg/6 hr PO for 2 days and it will suppress serum cortisol in patients with Cushing's disease (ACTH-secreting pituitary adenoma), however, it will fail to suppress serum cortisol in patients with Cushing's syndrome due to other causes (e.g. ectopic ACTH production, adrenal adenoma). It should, however, be noted that the high-dose dexamethasone suppression test is rarely used because it has a high false-positive rate. Following failure of suppression in a low-dose dexamethasone suppression test, the patient will be sent for inferior petrosal sinus sampling, which directly detects the output of ACTH from the pituitary gland.

13. B

The red reflex is the red reflection of light from the retina at the back of the eye. It can be seen using a fundoscope. Loss of the red reflex suggests that something is obscuring the retina. The best-known causes of loss of the red reflex are cataracts (opacification of the lens) and retinoblastoma (a rare form of cancer involving cells of the retina in children).

Herpes simplex keratitis is an infection of the cornea which causes a branched lesion on the cornea known as a 'dendritic ulcer'. It usually presents in adults due to reactivation of HSV, which has been lying dormant in the trigeminal nerve. Astigmatism is a refractive error of the focusing apparatus of the eye, caused by abnormalities of the cornea and lens. Conjunctivitis is inflammation of the conjunctiva, which causes itching and watering. Aniridia is the absence of the iris, which can be congenital or due to an injury.

14. E

A long history of abdominal pain, increased frequency and PR bleeding in a young person is suggestive of inflammatory bowel disease (IBD). The 'red ring' seen around the cornea is a feature of anterior uveitis, which is a common extra-intestinal manifestation of IBD. So, this patient is either presenting with Crohn's disease or ulcerative colitis (UC). There are some important points in the history that help distinguish between these. The abdominal pain tends to be diffuse in UC, whereas in Crohn's, it tends to be localised to the right iliac fossa. Urgency, diarrhoea and PR mucus are features of both diseases, but blood in the stool is more common in UC. Tenesmus is sometimes seen in UC. Furthermore, patients tend to be well in between attacks of UC, but fail to thrive in between attacks of Crohn's. This patient is presenting with bleeding and diffuse abdominal pain, making UC the most likely diagnosis. Mucosal ulcers, goblet cell depletion and crypt abscesses are classically seen in UC. Non-caseating granulomas are seen in Crohn's.

Eosinophilic infiltration occurs in eosinophilic gastroenteritis, an extremely rare condition characterised by eosinophilia of unknown cause. Eosinophils are part of the inflammatory process of UC, however, it is not the most appropriate answer. Villous atrophy and crypt hyperplasia are diagnostic of coeliac disease. Finally, high grade dysplasia and metaplastic columnar epithelium is describing Barrett's oesophagus — a condition characterised by metaplastic change of the lower oesophagus due to acid reflux.

15. C

Blurred vision and headaches are features of hyperviscosity. Other features include vertigo, seizures, hearing loss, ataxia and increased bleeding tendency. Polycythaemia (elevated haemoglobin concentration) is an important cause of hyperviscosity. Polycythaemia can be relative (normal red cell mass but reduced plasma volume) or absolute (increased red cell mass). Polycythaemia commonly presents with symptoms of hyperviscosity and pruritus (especially after a hot bath), which is likely to be the cause of this patient's scratch marks.

Polycythaemia can be further divided into primary or secondary poly-cythaemia. Polycythaemia rubra vera is a primary polycythaemia caused by clonal proliferation of myeloid stem cells. Secondary polycythaemia is caused by natural or artificial increases in erythropoietin (EPO) production. This increase in EPO production may be appropriate (e.g. in response to chronic hypoxia in COPD) or inappropriate (e.g. EPO abuse amongst athletes). This patient is an avid cyclist and has admitted to taking 'performance enhancers' (most likely EPO) to help improve his performance in his upcoming race. This practice is known as 'blood doping' and has resulted in this patient developing secondary polycythaemia.

16. D

Subclavian steal syndrome is a phenomenon in which stenosis of the subclavian artery proximal to the origin of the vertebral artery results in blood being 'stolen' from the brain by retrograde blood flow down the vertebral artery and into the arm. This tends to occur when there is an increased demand for blood in the arm (i.e. due to increased arm activity such as writing on a whiteboard). The retrograde blood flow down the vertebral artery means that less blood is flowing to the brain, resulting in blackout. The firm lump palpated in this patient's supraclavicular fossa is likely to be a cervical rib — an extra rib arising from the seven cervical vertebra — which can compress the subclavian artery. Other causes of subclavian artery stenosis include atherosclerosis and Takayasu's arteritis.

17. A

Nephrotic syndrome is a constellation of clinical features best described as a triad of proteinuria (>3.5 g/24 hrs), hypoalbuminaemia (<25 g/L) and oedema (often periorbital, peripheral or genital). Excretion of large amounts of protein in the urine means that there is less protein within the serum, therefore, there is less oncotic pressure drawing fluid back into the vasculature from the interstitium. This gives rise to oedema. Severe hyperlipidaemia is also associated with nephrotic syndrome. It is not a diagnosis in itself, so appropriate investigations are required to identify the underlying cause. Nephrotic syndrome may be caused by primary renal disease (e.g. minimal-change nephropathy, membranous nephropathy) or it may occur secondary to a systemic disorder (e.g. SLE, amyloidosis).

18. B

Guillain–Barré syndrome is an acute demyelinating polyneuropathy characterised by ascending symmetrical limb weakness and paraesthesia. In two-thirds of cases, symptoms occur a few days or weeks following an infection, with 30% of these infections being gastroenteritis caused by *Campylobacter jejuni*. Some other organisms that are often implicated in cases of Guillain–Barré syndrome include cytomegalovirus, EBV, HIV, influenza and travel infections such as Zika virus and dengue fever. Non-microbiological triggers include malignancy, surgery and post-vaccination (specifically the 1976 flu vaccine used against swine flu in the USA).

19. A

Antibiotics can be confusing. There are quite a lot of different drugs, and some of them sound quite similar and may have similar indications. However, most antibiotics tend to have one or two diseases that they are strongly associated with and most commonly used to treat. Community-acquired pneumonia (CAP) is most often caused by *Streptococcus pneumoniae* (70%). CAPs are treated with empirical antibiotics: co-amoxiclav (effective against *S. pneumoniae*) and clarithromycin (provides cover against atypical organisms).

Co-trimoxazole, a combination of trimethoprim and sulfamethoxazole, is used to treat *Pneumocystis jiroveci pneumonia* in HIV patients. It can also be used to treat some UTIs and respiratory tract infections. Metronidazole is effective against anaerobes, and, so, is used to treat several GI infections (e.g. *C. difficile* colitis), pelvic inflammatory disease and aspiration pneumonia. Flucloxacillin is a penicillin that is effective against Gram-positive bacteria (mainly *S. aureus*). It is often used to treat skin and soft tissue infections. Rifampicin and isoniazid are two of the four main drugs used in the treatment of TB.

20. A

Morphine sulphate is an opioid that is commonly used to provide analgesia in many scenarios, including the management of post-operative pain. Morphine is an effective analgesic but it causes several side-effects such as constipation, respiratory depression, nausea and drowsiness. It is important to monitor the bowel movements of patients on morphine, particularly if they are elderly, because it can lead to constipation, which, in turn, can cause confusion.

There are many drugs that can cause the other side-effects listed in the question, however, each of these side-effects has a particular drug or drug class that they are commonly associated with in SBAs: blurred vision = anti-muscarinic agents (e.g. atropine); cough = ACE inhibitors; tremor = beta-adrenergic receptor agonists (e.g. salbutamol); rash = ampicillin and amoxicillin in glandular fever.

21. E

Gout is an inflammatory arthritis caused by deposition of uric acid crystals within joints. The inflammation is most commonly localised to the metatarsophalangeal joint of the great toe (also known as podagra) and usually presents with excruciating monoarticular pain. Diagnosis is made by microscopy of a synovial fluid aspirate. Microscopy of synovial fluid in gout will show negatively birefringent, needle-shaped crystals. Pseudogout is another crystal arthropathy caused by the deposition of calcium pyrophosphate crystals and it typically affects the knees and wrists. In pseudogout, you will see positively birefringent, rhomboid-shaped crystals. Turbid synovial fluid with a high WCC is seen in septic arthritis.

22. D

Adrenal insufficiency tends to present, initially, with relatively vague symptoms (postural hypotension, abdominal pain, lethargy and weight loss). It is usually caused by autoimmune attack of the adrenal glands (most common in the UK) or tuberculosis (most common worldwide). Adrenal insufficiency results in reduced cortisol and aldosterone production by the adrenal glands. The reduced adrenal cortisol output leads to increased ACTH production by the pituitary gland, via negative feedback. POMC is the precursor of ACTH, which also produces alpha-MSH (melanocyte-stimulating hormone) as a by-product. High levels of ACTH in adrenal insufficiency are, therefore, accompanied by high levels of alpha-MSH — this causes increased skin pigmentation, especially of the buccal mucosa and palmar creases. Vitiligo is characterised by autoimmune attack of melanocytes leading to patches of skin depigmentation. It is sometimes found in patients with adrenal insufficiency as autoimmune diseases tend to come hand-in-hand. A short synacthen test involves administering a synthetic ACTH (synacthen) and observing the cortisol response. A cortisol level <550 nmol/L measured 30 mins after synacthen administration is suggestive of adrenal insufficiency.

A full blood count is requested for a vast variety of reasons and may be performed in this patient to check whether anaemia is contributing to her lethargy, however, it is not the most appropriate investigation in this scenario. Fasting blood glucose is used to diagnose diabetes mellitus. An ECG may be used to check for rhythm disturbances that could cause faintness and loss of consciousness.

23. A

Change in bowel habit, PR bleeding and weight loss in an elderly person raises suspicion of colorectal cancer. The presentation of colorectal cancer can vary depending on the location of the tumour. Left-sided colorectal cancer tends to present earlier with a change in bowel habit and PR bleeding, whereas right-sided tends to present later with abdominal pain and symptoms of anaemia (e.g. shortness of breath, fatigue). There is a degree of overlap between these presentations as left-sided colorectal cancers are also associated with symptoms of anaemia. The patient's description of not feeling empty after defecation is referred to as 'tenesmus'. It is caused by the presence of space-occupying lesions in the rectum (e.g. cancer). Colorectal cancer most commonly occurs in the rectum (27%) followed by the sigmoid colon (20%) and caecum (14%). A DRE should be performed (which, in this patient, may reveal a low-lying rectal mass) and serum carcinoembryonic antigen (CEA — the most specific tumour marker for colorectal cancer) should be measured. Ultimately, a definitive diagnosis will be made based on the results of a colonoscopy and biopsy.

Don't get caught out by the enlargement of Virchow's node (Troisier's sign) described in this SBA. Although this is most often associated with gastric cancer, it can also be found in other abdominal malignancies. Gastric cancer is also more likely to present with dyspepsia, vomiting, early satiety, bloating and melaena. The presentation of pancreatic cancer given in SBAs is typically in accordance with Courvoisier's law: *Painless jaundice in the presence of a palpable gallbladder is unlikely to be due to gallstones* (i.e. it is more likely to be due to cancer).

24. E

The circle of Willis is a ring of arteries within the brain formed by the joining of branches of the internal carotid arteries (anterior cerebral arteries (ACA) and middle cerebral arteries (MCA)) and the basilar artery (which is a continuation of the two vertebral arteries). The posterior cerebral artery (PCA) arises in between the MCA and the basilar artery. The cerebral arteries supply different parts of the brain and, therefore, cause different signs and symptoms if occluded. This is summarised in the table below:

Artery	Region of brain supplied	Presentation
Anterior cerebral artery	Medial aspect of the frontal and parietal lobes	Behavioural changes Weakness of contralateral leg > arm Mild sensory deficit
Middle cerebral artery	Lateral aspect of the frontal, temporal and parietal lobes Subcortical structures (e.g. basal ganglia, internal capsule)	Contralateral hemiparesis of face > arm > leg aphasia Hemisensory deficits Loss of contralateral half of visual field
Posterior cerebral artery	Occipital lobes Inferior and medical portion of temporal lobes	Loss of contralateral half of visual filed Sensory deficit Visual agnosia Prosopagnosia

This patient is experiencing expressive aphasia, right-sided weakness which is worst in the face and arms, and right homonymous hemianopia. This is consistent with a left MCA occlusion.

25. C

Hyponatraemia is a very common electrolyte abnormality. Sodium is one of the major solutes in the extracellular fluid compartment and it is a measure of fluid status rather than salt concentration. Hyponatraemia indicates a dilution of the extracellular fluid due to an excess of water. Symptoms depend on the degree of hyponatraemia and the speed of onset. In the majority of cases, hyponatraemia is mild (130–135 mmol/L) and asymptomatic. Moderate hyponatraemia (125–130 mmol/L) may cause non-specific symptoms, such as headaches, nausea, lethargy, and muscle cramps. Severe hyponatraemia is defined as serum sodium <120 mmol/L and is associated with neurological symptoms such as seizures, hallucinations, confusion and memory loss. Hyponatraemia can be fatal if the serum sodium drops acutely over 24–28 hrs as this can lead to cerebral oedema, coning and respiratory arrest.

This patient is severely hyponatraemic and, therefore, would be expected to be symptomatic. As he is asymptomatic, it is likely that this is a case of pseudohyponatraemia — the serum sodium concentration is normal but it is erroneously reported as being low. This is due to the presence of high levels of lipids or proteins in the sample, which dilutes the aqueous component of the extracellular compartment thereby decreasing the apparent sodium concentration.

26. E

Left lower lobe collapse leads to a leftward tracheal deviation and the edge of the collapsed left lower lobe forms, what looks like, a second heart border. The contrast between the border of the collapsed left lower lobe and the heart shadow creates a 'sail' shape. Right upper lobe collapse produces 'Golden S sign' because the outline of the collapsed lobe looks like a reversed 'S'.

27. A

The cardinal features of bowel obstruction are vomiting, colicky abdominal pain, constipation (described as 'absolute' if no flatus or faeces has been passed) and abdominal distention. Vomiting occurs earlier in small bowel obstruction and pain tends to be felt higher up in the abdomen when compared with large bowel obstruction, in which the pain is more constant and vomiting is a less prominent feature. An abdominal X-ray is the first-line investigation, which will show dilated loops of bowel. The normal diameters of different parts of the intestines can be remembered using the 3/6/9 rule: 3 cm = small bowel, 6 cm = large bowel, 9 cm = caecum. Previous abdominal surgery is a significant feature of this history as it means that this patient may have adhesions. Adhesions are fibrous bands that form between the intestines and the peritoneum and can cause bowel obstruction, typically after abdominal surgery. Adhesions are the most common cause of bowel obstruction in the Western world. Other common causes include tumours, constipation and hernias.

Bowel obstruction is a surgical emergency and it is managed using 'drip and suck'. This involves gaining IV access to administer fluids (drip) and inserting an NG tube to aspirate gastric contents (suck) and decompress the bowel. In 75% of cases, adhesions resolve spontaneously with conservative management. Patients must be assessed regularly to look for signs of peritonism (indicative of a strangulated or perforated bowel). Surgery is considered in patients who have not improved with conservative management after 48 hrs, have signs of peritonism, a palpable mass or a virgin abdomen (no previous surgery).

28. E

When young people are diagnosed with hypertension, it is important to think of the secondary causes. Coarctation of the aorta is a congenital condition characterised by narrowing of the aorta, and it is a well-known cause of secondary hypertension. On examination, if the narrowing occurs proximal to the left subclavian artery, it will cause radio-radial delay, whereas if it occurs distal to the left subclavian artery it will cause radio-femoral delay.

Conn's syndrome, also known as primary hyperaldosteronism, is the excess production of aldosterone by the adrenal glands. Renal artery stenosis refers to narrowing of the renal artery. Both are causes of secondary hypertension. An aortic dissection occurs when a tear in the tunica intima of the aorta allows blood to surge into the aortic wall and cause a separation between the inner and outer tunica media, creating a false lumen. It presents with a sudden 'tearing' chest pain that may radiate to the back. An aortic transection is when the aorta tears due to trauma. This is often fatal and is commonly associated with death due to road traffic accidents.

29. A

Meralgia paraesthetica is numbness, pain or paraesthesia affecting an area of skin on the outside of the thigh caused by injury to the lateral femoral cutaneous nerve. It can be caused by weight gain resulting in gradually tightening belts or trouser waistbands. Therefore, patients are often advised to lose weight and wear looser clothing. NSAIDs may also be used to help deal with the pain.

30. D

Primary biliary cirrhosis (PBC) is T-cell mediated autoimmune inflammation and destruction of the intrahepatic biliary ducts. Patients are often asymptomatic with a diagnosis being made due to abnormal LFTs (persistently elevated ALP, GGT and mild transaminitis). Symptoms may include extreme lethargy, right upper quadrant pain, pruritus and jaundice and signs include jaundice, xanthelesma and xanthomata (due to increased cholesterol levels), hepatomegaly and splenomegaly. PBC presents relatively similarly to primary sclerosing cholangitis (PSC). The presence of anti-mitochondrial antibodies is a distinguishing feature of PBC with over 90% of PBC patients testing positive. PBC is associated with other autoimmune conditions, such as rheumatoid arthritis, Sjögren's syndrome (hence the dry, itchy eyes), coeliac disease and scleroderma.

Paper 3

Questions

1. A 53-year-old woman has been suffering from recurrent painful episodes affecting her face — mainly her right cheek. She describes the pain as being extremely intense, sharp and sudden, like an 'electric shock'. It usually lasts for a few seconds before subsiding. The pain often occurs when she brushes her teeth. What is the most likely diagnosis?

   A Giant cell arteritis
   B Trigeminal neuralgia
   C Ramsay Hunt syndrome
   D Shingles
   E Cluster headache

2. A 21-year-old woman visits the GP complaining of a 2-month history of bloating and watery diarrhoea. She adds that she often has to rush to the toilet. During the consultation, she starts furiously itching her elbows. On examination, there is a blistering, papulovesicular rash covering both elbows. What is the most likely diagnosis?

   A Inflammatory bowel disease
   B Coeliac disease
   C Gastroenteritis

    D Irritable bowel syndrome

    E Ischaemic colitis

3. Which of the following is NOT a chest X-ray feature of heart failure?

    A Kerley B lines

    B Upper lobe diversion

    C Cardiomegaly

    D Pleural effusion

    E Air bronchograms

4. A 71-year-old man is referred to the oncology clinic having suffered from hip pain, constipation and abdominal pain for the past few months. He has also noticed that he is having to urinate more frequently than usual, and, consequently, he is always extremely thirsty. A full blood count and U&Es are requested:

Hb = 105 g/L (130–175)

MCV = 106 fl (76–96)

Platelets = 120 $\times$ 10^9/L (150–400 $\times$ 10^9)

Creatinine = 125 μmol/L (baseline: 72 μmol/L (3 months ago))

The oncologist requests a blood film. Considering the most likely diagnosis, what would you expect to see on this patient's blood film?

    A Rouleaux formation

    B Schistocytes

    C Granulocytes with absent granulation and hyposegmented nuclei

    D Dacrocytes

    E Smear cells

5. A 56-year-old woman, of Somalian origin, presents with a 2-month history of haemoptysis. She has also noticed some weight loss during this time and complains that she is having to change her bed sheets more often than usual as they are often drenched with sweat in the morning. Examination reveals painless cervical lymphadenopathy

and tender, purple lumps on her shins. A CXR reveals an area of consolidation in the right upper lobe. Which investigation should be performed next in order to establish a diagnosis?

    A Bronchoalveolar lavage
    B Chest CT scan
    C Sputum sample for acid-fast bacilli
    D Bronchoscopy and biopsy
    E Mantoux test

6. Which type of urinary tract stone is most common?

    A Magnesium ammonium phosphate
    B Calcium oxalate
    C Cysteine
    D Urate
    E Hydroxyapatite

7. A 62-year-old man presents with severe, acute epigastric pain with nausea and vomiting. The pain radiates to the back and improves when sitting forward. It started 4 days ago, but the patient assumed it was indigestion and refused to come to hospital. On examination, there is epigastric tenderness and ecchymoses over the periumbilical area and flank. The patient drinks in moderation and has not had any alcohol recently. Serum amylase is 600 U/L (<140). Which investigation should be performed to confirm the diagnosis?

    A ERCP
    B Abdominal CT scan
    C Abdominal X-ray
    D Abdominal ultrasound
    E MRCP

8. A 39-year-old carpenter is brought into A&E having fallen from a 3rd floor balcony. He landed on his head and has been unconscious since the incident. An intracranial haemorrhage is suspected and an urgent

CT scan is requested. The patient's vital signs are recorded: BP = 195/120 mm Hg; HR = 47 bpm (60–100). His breathing also appears to be irregular — shallow breaths interspersed with periods of apnoea. What is the name given to this phenomenon?

   A Kussmaul sign
   B Cushing's reflex
   C Beck's triad
   D Charcot's triad
   E Baroreceptor reflex

9. A 46-year-old woman visits A&E complaining of a fever and episodes of shivering. She returned from Nigeria 2 weeks ago and confesses that she was not very compliant with her antimalarial medication. Therefore, malaria is suspected. Which investigation should be performed to diagnose malaria?

   A Thick and thin blood films
   B Blood cultures
   C Heterophile antibody test
   D Enzyme-linked Immunosorbent Assay (ELISA)
   E Urinalysis

10. A patient suffering an acute exacerbation of COPD has become hypoxic with an SaO_2 of 83%. He requires administration of oxygen at a tightly regulated concentration. Which of the following methods of administering oxygen would be most appropriate?

   A Nasal cannula
   B Hudson face mask
   C Venturi mask
   D Non-rebreathing mask
   E BiPAP

11. A 48-year-old man has been suffering from frequent urination for the past 5 months. He has been going to the toilet around 10 times per day

and he has been drinking excessive volumes of water. He has also been constipated for the past month with vague 'tummy pains' and complains of joint pain in his hands. A blood test is requested, which shows:

Na$^+$: 137 mmol/L (135–145)
K$^+$: 4.6 mmol/L (3.5–5)
Ca^{2+}: 3.0 mmol/L (2.2–2.6)
ALP: 197 iU/L (30–150)
PTH: 9.6 SI units (1.1–6.8)

What is the most likely diagnosis?

    A Vitamin D Toxicosis
    B Parathyroid Adenoma
    C Paget's Disease
    D Malignancy
    E Milk-Alkali Syndrome

12. A 61-year-old male comes to A&E complaining of chest pain and mentions that he can feel his heart 'pumping out of his chest'. An ECG shows regular broad complex tachycardia, with no P waves. His blood pressure is 124/87 mm Hg. How should this patient be treated?

    A Defibrillation
    B DC cardioversion
    C Amiodarone
    D Adenosine
    E Atropine

13. A 30-year-old man presents to his GP complaining of a swollen scrotum, which he first noticed 3 weeks ago. He adds that the swelling feels like a 'bag of worms', and, despite being a little uncomfortable, it is not painful. On examination, the patient's scrotum looks normal when he is supine, however, the left hemiscrotum becomes swollen

when he stands up. The GP can get above the swelling and distinguish it from the testicle. What is the most likely diagnosis?

    A Indirect inguinal hernia
    B Direct inguinal hernia
    C Hydrocoele
    D Varicocoele
    E Epididymal cyst

14. A 74-year-old woman is brought to A&E having suffered several violent bouts of vomiting. On examination, she is clearly distressed and has a massively distended abdomen. When questioned, she struggles to answer but complains of generalised abdominal pain and mentions that she hasn't passed any faeces or flatus since the pain began. Bowel obstruction is suspected and an AXR is requested. The AXR shows a massively distended loop of large bowel which looks like an embryo. What is the most likely cause of this bowel obstruction?

    A Colorectal cancer
    B Sigmoid volvulus
    C Caecal volvulus
    D Adhesions
    E Femoral hernia

15. A 36-year-old female presents to the GP complaining that the nail bed of her ring finger has detached and she is worried that the same is happening to her other finger nails. The GP suspects onycholysis. Which of the following diseases is most commonly associated with onycholysis?

    A SLE
    B Psoriasis
    C Thyrotoxicosis
    D Hyperlipidaemia
    E Polycythaemia rubra vera

16. A 72-year-old man has recently suffered a stroke. He has recovered well and appears to have regained much of his physical strength, however, his speech has changed quite considerably. His daughter says that he will talk the same amount as he always did but his sentences will not make any sense, and he doesn't seem to notice. When asked to describe what he did this morning, he responds: 'The bugle fidget and that I played tractor to you before'. Damage to which part of the brain is likely to manifest in this way?

 A Wernicke's area
 B Broca's area
 C Arcuate fasciculus
 D Hippocampus
 E Amygdala

17. An inpatient on the surgical ward is recovering after having a kidney stone removed. A routine blood test is performed which shows the following results:

 Na$^+$: 135 mmol/L (135–145)
 K$^+$: 8.7 mmol/L (3.5–6.0)
 Ca^{2+}: 0.2 mmol/L (2.2–2.6)

An ECG is performed which shows no obvious abnormalities.

Given the above information, what should be the next step in the management of this patient?

 A Urgently draw another blood sample
 B 10 mL 10% calcium gluconate
 C 20 mL 20% calcium gluconate
 D 50 mL 50% dextrose + 10 U insulin
 E IV salbutamol

18. What are the 'B symptoms' of lymphoma?

    A Fever, Lymphadenopathy, Rigors
    B Fever, Night sweats, Weight loss
    C Recurrent infections, Anaemia, Easy bruising
    D Night sweats, Pruritus, Weight loss
    E Lymphadenopathy, Weight loss, Loss of appetite

19. A 40-year-old teacher has recently heard several distressing comments about how flushed she is looking. On examination, she has very red cheeks and a loud S1 with a mid-diastolic murmur is heard over the apex when the patient is in the left lateral position. What is the most likely diagnosis?

    A Mitral stenosis
    B Mitral regurgitation
    C Aortic stenosis
    D Aortic regurgitation
    E Tricuspid regurgitation

20. A 59-year-old female presents with epigastric pain that gets worse a few hours after eating. The patient has taken ibuprofen every day for the past 2 years for her chronic back pain. A urea breath test is negative. What is the most appropriate treatment option for this patient?

    A Stop ibuprofen and give omeprazole
    B Stop ibuprofen and give ranitidine
    C Give amoxicillin, metronidazole and pantoprazole
    D Give lifestyle advice and arrange to see the patient in 3 months
    E Oral steroids

21. A 58-year-old woman presents to her GP with a 5-month history of worsening shortness of breath on exertion. She has also lost about 3 kg in weight and has experienced a dry cough. She has never smoked before and has a past medical history of rheumatoid arthritis, which was diagnosed 15 years ago. On examination, her fingers are

clubbed and fine inspiratory crackles are heard bilaterally across the lower lung zones. What is the most likely diagnosis?

    A COPD
    B Lung cancer
    C Bronchiectasis
    D Pulmonary fibrosis
    E Tuberculosis

22. A 38-year-old woman has been experiencing palpitations, sweating and diarrhoea for the past week. Before these symptoms began, she was on sick leave for 3 days with a fever, sore throat and cough. During the consultation, she appears to be very anxious with a slight tremor in her hands. Vital signs: HR = 114, Temp = 38.6°C. A thyroid examination reveals a warm, tender and slightly enlarged thyroid gland. A thyroid uptake scan is requested. What would you expect to see?

    A Diffuse uptake throughout an enlarged gland
    B No uptake
    C Multinodular gland with multiple hot nodules
    D Multinodular gland with a single hot nodule
    E Diffuse uptake with a single cold nodule

23. A 24-year-old waitress presents to her GP after noticing a small, firm lump in her left breast. She first noticed the lump 1 week ago and is unsure about whether it has grown. She reports no nipple discharge or skin changes over the breast. Examination reveals a 1 × 2 cm lump in the upper outer quadrant of the left breast with no axillary lymphadenopathy. She is worried because her grandmother died of breast cancer. What is the next most appropriate step in the management of this patient?

    A Urgent mammogram
    B Urgent ultrasound scan
    C Urgent CT scan
    D Arrange elective mastectomy
    E Arrange elective wide local excision

24. A 73-year-old man was watching TV with his family, 2 hrs ago, when his speech suddenly became slurred and he lost the ability to grip the remote control. His son, who accompanied him to A&E, noticed that the left half of his father's face drooped during this episode. His symptoms eventually subsided after around 15 mins and he claims that he feels back to normal, albeit slightly shaken by his ordeal. What is the first step in his management?

    A Administer aspirin
    B Thrombolysis
    C CT head scan
    D ECG
    E Carotid endarterectomy

25. A 9-year-old girl is brought to see her GP, by her father, because she has been complaining of pain in her knees and ankles and a tummy ache, which began yesterday. Urinalysis is positive for blood and protein. On examination, small purple spots are seen on her buttocks and her knees feel warm and swollen. Her father adds that, 2 weeks ago, she took time off school because of the flu. What is the most likely diagnosis?

    A Post-infectious glomerulonephritis
    B Immune thrombocytopenic purpura
    C Disseminated intravascular coagulation
    D Henoch-Schönlein purpura
    E Minimal change glomerulonephritis

26. A 64-year-old woman presents with severe left iliac fossa pain with nausea and vomiting. She adds that she has had a few episodes of rectal bleeding recently where the blood has coated the stools. She admits to eating a lot of fast food and having a low-fibre diet. She has not noticed any weight loss. Her left iliac fossa is tender on

palpation and blood is found on DRE. What is the most likely diagnosis?

    A Gastroenteritis
    B Diverticulitis
    C Angiodysplasia
    D Colorectal carcinoma
    E Inflammatory bowel disease

27. Which of the following organisms is responsible for causing whooping cough?

    A *Bordatella pertussis*
    B *Treponema pallidum*
    C *Cryptosporidium*
    D *Mycoplasma pneumoniae*
    E *Yersinia pestis*

28. A 59-year-old man is brought to A&E by his daughter after having collapsed at home. He has very little recollection of the incident — one minute he was doing the dishes, and next minute he was lying on his back on the floor. He has no history of recent head trauma and mentions that he felt 'absolutely fine' when he regained consciousness. An ECG is performed showing bradycardia (36 bpm) and dissociation between the p waves and QRS complexes. A diagnosis of complete heart block is made. What might be seen on close inspection of his JVP?

    A Large V waves
    B Cannon A waves
    C Kussmaul sign
    D Raised JVP with absent pulsation
    E Slow Y descent

29. A 36-year-old supermarket manager has been suffering from chronic back pain and stiffness. He first saw his GP about this matter 6 months ago and was given paracetamol, however, the pain worsened and has started affecting his job. He finds restocking the shelves particularly difficult as it requires repetitively bending down and picking up products. He mentions that the pain and stiffness is worst in the morning and gradually gets better with activity. What is the most likely diagnosis?

    A Ankylosing spondylitis
    B Lumbar disc herniation
    C Osteoarthritis
    D Muscle strain
    E Vertebral fracture

30. A 69-year-old man is recovering in the inpatient respiratory ward having been diagnosed with pneumonia yesterday. A right-sided pleural effusion is identified on the chest X-ray. Which of the following findings on clinical examination of the right lung base, would be most consistent with a right-sided pleural effusion?

    A Resonant percussion note, increased vocal resonance, vesicular breathing
    B Resonant percussion note, reduced vocal resonance, reduced breath sounds
    C Dull percussion note, increased vocal resonance, bronchial breathing
    D Dull percussion note, decreased vocal resonance, reduced breath sounds
    E Dull percussion note, decreased vocal resonance, vesicular breathing

Answers

1. B

Trigeminal neuralgia is an intense neuropathic pain affecting one or more branches of the trigeminal nerve. It is thought to be caused by compression of the trigeminal nerve, although the exact mechanism is not fully understood. It is associated with multiple sclerosis. It typically presents with recurrent episodes of sharp, stabbing facial pain which can last seconds to minutes. It can be triggered by skin contact, brushing your teeth and shaving.

Shingles refers, broadly, to the reactivation of varicella zoster virus. Ramsay Hunt syndrome is a type of shingles caused by reactivation of varicella zoster in the geniculate ganglion of the facial nerve. It presents with facial nerve palsy, altered taste, dry eyes/mouth and a vesicular rash in the ear canal. Cluster headaches are recurrent, severe, unilateral headaches, typically located around one eye that occurs daily (i.e. in clusters) over a period of weeks. Patients also often experience eye symptoms (e.g. lacrimation, conjunctival injection, eyelid swelling).

2. B

Bloating, diarrhoea and urgency in a young person can be caused by inflammatory bowel disease (IBD), irritable bowel syndrome (IBS), coeliac disease and gastroenteritis. This patient has a long history of symptoms, making acute illnesses like gastroenteritis less likely. IBD and ischaemic colitis are also less likely as these typically cause bloody diarrhoea. Furthermore, ischaemic colitis usually occurs in elderly patients. The blistering, papulovesicular rash covering her elbows is likely to be dermatitis herpetiformis, which is an extra-GI manifestation of coeliac disease. This, coupled with the GI symptoms described, makes coeliac disease the most likely diagnosis.

Coeliac disease is an inflammatory condition caused by intolerance to gluten, found in grains and starches, such as wheat, rye and barley. Gluten consumption triggers an immunological reaction in the small bowel, mediated by T cells, which leads to the disruption of the structure and function of the mucosal lining. This ultimately leads to malabsorption, malnutrition and anaemia (due to iron deficiency). Commonly experienced symptoms include diarrhoea, steatorrhoea (pale, greasy and offensive smelling stools), weight loss, crampy abdominal pain, bloating, flatulence, urgency and recurrent mouth ulcers. The first-line investigation is serology to look for tissue transglutaminase antibodies, anti-endomysial antibodies and anti-gliadin antibodies, all of which will be elevated in coeliac disease. A definitive diagnosis is established based on the findings of OGD and duodenal biopsy. The classic histological appearance of bowel affected by coeliac disease is the presence of *'subtotal villous atrophy with crypt hyperplasia'*.

3. E

The chest X-ray findings of heart failure can be remembered using the mnemonic **ABCDE**: **A**lveolar oedema, Kerley **B** lines, **C**ardiomegaly, upper lobe **D**iversion and pleural **E**ffusion. Air bronchograms refer to the appearance of bronchi (which are radiolucent) that are made visible when something other than air is filling the surrounding alveoli — such as pus in pneumonia, fluid in pulmonary oedema and fibrosed tissue in interstitial lung disease.

4. A

This patient's presenting symptoms should make you think of the *'stones, bones, abdominal groans, thrones and psychiatric overtones'* of hypercalcaemia. In addition, the rise in creatinine suggests that this patient has developed acute renal failure. He also has macrocytic anaemia — low Hb and high MCV. To summarise, this features of hyper-**C**alcaemia, **R**enal failure, **A**naemia and **B**one pain constitutes the main features of multiple myeloma, remembered as '**CRAB**'. Multiple myeloma is a haematological malignancy characterised by an excessive proliferation of plasma cells. It causes bone lesions (and hence, hypercalcaemia) and the production of monoclonal immunoglobulins. Rouleaux are stacks of red cells seen on a blood film, which form due to the high concentration of plasma proteins (e.g. immunoglobulins) and give rise to the high ESR.

Schistocytes, also known as red cell fragments, are an indicator of intra-vascular haemolysis. Granulocytes with absent granulation and hyposeg-mented nuclei are found in myelodysplastic syndrome. Dacrocytes are teardrop-shaped cells seen in myelofibrosis. Smear cells are seen in chronic lymphocytic leukaemia.

5. C

The clinical scenario described by this SBA is typical of tuberculosis — a woman from a TB-endemic country presenting with haemoptysis, weight loss, night sweats, cervical lymphadenopathy and erythema nodosum. This is further supported by the presence of an area of consolidation on the CXR. N.B. TB tends to affect the upper lobes. The CXR may also show hilar lymphadenopathy. The best investigation to establish a diagno-sis is a sputum sample, which should be tested for the presence of acid-fast bacilli using Ziehl–Neelsen stain. A sputum culture should be requested at the same time; however, this can take up to 6 weeks to pro-duce results. The Mantoux test is a technique in which an intradermal injection of tuberculin purified protein derivative is administered and a reaction producing a raised, hardened area around the injection site after 72 hrs suggests that the patient has previously been exposed to TB. Although it can identify patients who have been exposed to TB, it does not distinguish between active and latent TB.

6. B

Type of urinary tract stone in order of prevalence:

> Calcium oxalate – 75%
> Magnesium ammonium phosphate (struvite) – 15%
> Urate – 5%
> Hydroxyapatite – 5%
> Cysteine – 1%

7. D

Transabdominal ultrasound scan is the first investigation used for sus-pected pancreatitis as it is inexpensive, can be performed at the bedside and allows visualisation of the biliary tree. Ultrasound can also show pancreatic inflammation, calcification and free fluid. CT is useful for staging pancreatitis and detecting complications. MRCP may be used instead of CT in patients with renal insufficiency who cannot tolerate IV contrast. ERCP has therapeutic potential (e.g. stent placement, sphincterotomy), however, it is only performed in patients with confirmed gallstones. Abdominal X-ray may help by showing a sentinel loop of bowel (localised ileus caused by intra-abdominal inflammation). Pancreatitis should not be excluded on the basis of mildly elevated or normal amylase because amylase has a half-life of 10–12 hours, so it will return to normal levels after about 3–5 days.

8. B

The Cushing's reflex is a physiological response to raised intracranial pressure, characterised by a triad of high blood pressure, bradycardia and irregular breathing. This patient's raised ICP is likely to be due to cerebral oedema or an intracranial haemorrhage following head trauma.

Kussmaul sign is a paradoxical rise in JVP on inspiration, which occurs in patients with impaired right ventricular filling (e.g. constrictive pericarditis, restrictive cardiomyopathy). Beck's triad refers to three signs seen in patients with cardiac tamponade: raised JVP, muffled heart sounds and low blood pressure. Charcot's triad is the three main features of ascending cholangitis: right upper quadrant pain, jaundice and fever with rigors. The baroreceptor reflex is the homeostatic mechanism that maintains a constant blood pressure.

9. A

Malaria is caused by infection with the protozoan *Plasmodium* of which there are five main species: *P. falciparum, P. vivax, P. malariae, P. ovale* and *P. knowlesi*. *P. falciparum* is responsible for causing the greatest number of deaths. *Plasmodium* is transmitted by the bite of the female *Anopheles* mosquito. It goes on to infect red blood cells and replicate intracellularly. Malaria should be suspected in travellers from malaria-endemic countries who have been experiencing cyclical episodes of shivering and chills followed by fever and sweating. Malaria is diagnosed following the microscopic analysis of blood films. There are two main types of blood films: thin and thick. Thin films preserve the appearance of the parasites allowing species identification. Thick films screen a larger volume of blood allowing higher sensitivity when picking up low-level infections.

10. C

Patients with COPD lose their hypercapnic drive to breathe, therefore, they become reliant on their hypoxic response to maintain neural respiratory drive. So, carefully titrated oxygen concentrations must be given to patients with acute exacerbations of COPD (usually aiming for SaO$_2$ 88–92%) to preserve the hypoxic drive to breathe. Venturi masks offer the best precision when delivering oxygen.

Nasal cannulae are patient-friendly, however, it is relatively imprecise and can only administer a relatively low flow of oxygen. Hudson face masks deliver a variable amount of oxygen and are much less precise than Venturi masks. Non-rebreathing masks are useful for delivering a high concentration of oxygen (60–100%), however, they too are imprecise. BiPAP (bilevel positive airway pressure) is a form of non-invasive ventilation used to treat respiratory acidosis and obstructive sleep apnoea.

11. B

The classic *'stones, bones, abdominal groans, thrones and psychiatric overtones'* summarises the key features of hypercalcaemia: Kidney stones, bone and joint pain, urinary frequency (commode = throne), vague abdominal pain and psychiatric disturbance. There are two main hormones that are responsible for increasing serum Ca^{2+} levels: Parathyroid hormone (PTH) and 1,25-dihydroxy vitamin D3 (calcitriol). PTH is produced by the parathyroid gland (found embedded in the thyroid gland). Calcitriol is produced using a combination of UV light, dietary vitamin D and enzymes in the liver and kidneys. PTH follows a simple feedback loop with serum Ca^{2+} concentration. When Ca^{2+} is high (as in this patient), PTH should be low — so, if the PTH level is elevated or even within the 'normal range', it is considered abnormal. Hyperparathyroidism is most often caused by parathyroid hyperplasia and parathyroid adenomas.

Hypercalcaemia of malignancy is a condition that results from the release of calcium from bone metastases or from the paraneoplastic effect of PTH-related peptides, which can be released by cancer cells and mimic the action of PTH. In hypercalcaemia of malignancy, the Ca^{2+} level will be raised but the PTH feedback loop will be intact, so the PTH level will be low. Paget's disease is a disorder of bone metabolism that does not affect serum Ca^{2+} levels. Milk-Alkali syndrome is a rare condition caused by the ingestion of too much calcium and alkali (e.g. from dietary supplements used to prevent osteoporosis).

12. C

This is a case of ventricular tachycardia (VT), a type of broad complex tachycardia. There are many causes of VT including coronary artery disease, valvular disease, electrolyte imbalances (e.g. low Mg^{2+}) and long QT syndrome. As this patient is haemodynamically stable, IV amiodarone should be given first. Where possible treat the underlying cause (e.g. correct electrolyte imbalances). If this patient has no palpable pulse (i.e. pulseless VT), he should be treated according to the Advanced Life Support (ALS) guidelines:

1. Defibrillate
2. Perform CPR for 2 mins and then defibrillate again
3. Administer IV adrenaline after the 2nd defibrillation is delivered, and repeat every 3–5 mins
4. If the abnormal rhythm persists after the 3rd defibrillation, administer IV amiodarone.

Atropine used to be part of the treatment guidelines for cardiac arrest but has since been removed. Adenosine is used to terminate supraventricular tachycardia.

13. D

A varicocoele is a scrotal mass formed by the dilation of the veins of the pampiniform plexus. 80–90% of varicocoeles occur on the left because of the angle at which the left testicular vein meets the renal vein and increased reflux from compression of the renal vein. Varicocoeles are usually asymptomatic, however, they can cause a sense of scrotal heaviness. On examination, the lump is often described as feeling like a 'bag of worms'. Varicocoeles are reducible so the patient must be standing when examined and actions that increase intra-abdominal pressure (e.g. Valsalva manoeuvre, coughing) can increase the dilatation. They are associated with infertility.

The GP will not be able to get above an inguinal hernia. It would not be possible to distinguish the swelling from the testicle in a hydrocoele. Epididymal cysts will not reduce when lying down and it would cause a smooth, fluctuant swelling rather than a 'bag of worms'.

14. C

Bowel obstruction usually presents with acute generalised abdominal pain, nausea, vomiting and absolute constipation. The most common causes of bowel obstruction are tumours, adhesions, volvuli and hernias. Abdominal X-rays (AXR) are often requested in cases of bowel obstruction because they can help distinguish between large bowel obstruction (distended bowel around outside of the abdomen, with haustra) and small bowel obstruction (distended bowel in the middle of the abdomen, with valvulae conniventes). A volvulus is formed when the stomach or a loop of bowel twists on its mesentery, leading to strangulation and obstruction. It is more likely to happen to parts of the bowel that hang loosely on its mesentery (i.e. sigmoid and caecum). A caecal volvulus produces a gas bubble on AXR that looks like an embryo and, hence, is called 'embryo sign'.

A sigmoid volvulus produces a gas bubble in the shape of a coffee bean — 'coffee bean sign'. Colorectal cancer, femoral hernias and adhesions will show the classic features of bowel obstruction on AXR but the appearance is variable and they are not associated with looking like an embryo. SBAs in which adhesions are the cause of bowel obstruction are likely to mention previous abdominal surgery — a major risk factor for the formation of adhesions.

15. B

Onycholysis is a common nail condition characterised by painless separation of the fingernail or toenail from the nailbed. There are many causes of onycholysis — some examples can be remembered using the mnemonic **DR PITHS**:

- **D**rugs (e.g. tetracyclines, oral contraceptive and diabetes drugs)
- **R**eactive arthritis, Reiter's syndrome (rare)
- **P**soriasis
- **I**nfection (especially fungal)
- **T**rauma
- **H**yper- and Hypothyroidism (rare)
- **S**arcoidosis, Scleroderma (rare)

16. A

Damage to Wernicke's area results in the inability to understand language, however, patients will be able to produce fluent, but non-sensical, speech (as described in this patient). Broca's area, located in the frontal lobe of the dominant hemisphere, is responsible for speech production. Damage to Broca's area leads to an inability to produce fluent speech, despite intact understanding of language.

The arcuate fasciculus connects Wernicke's and Broca's areas. Lesions of the arcuate fasciculus results in intact language comprehension and fluent speech production; however, speech repetition is poor. The hippocampus, a component of the limbic system, is responsible for memory and learning. The amygdala, also in the limbic system, is a component of the fight or flight response.

17. A

This is a classic trap that many students will fall into. Treating hyperkalaemia with 10 mL 10% calcium gluconate is one of those typical buzzword SBAs that all medical students love, but make sure that you read the question properly! Drawing blood too fast can lead to red cell lysis, releasing all the intracellular potassium into the sample. This is a common cause of erroneously high potassium levels. In this circumstance, another set of bloods should be taken urgently. Furthermore, a potassium >6 mmol/L is very likely to cause ECG changes and a calcium of 0.2 mmol/L is incompatible with life!

18. B

'B symptoms' of lymphoma refers to fever, night sweats and weight loss. The presence of B symptoms in a patient with lymphoma is a prognostic indicator of advanced disease exerting systemic effects.

19. A

The examination findings are consistent with mitral stenosis. Different murmurs correspond to different valvular problems as follows:

Aortic and Pulmonary Stenosis — Ejection Systolic Murmur
Aortic and Pulmonary Regurgitation — Early Diastolic Murmur
Mitral and Tricuspid Stenosis — Mid-Diastolic Murmur
Mitral and Tricuspid Regurgitation — Pansystolic Murmur

Right-sided (i.e. tricuspid and pulmonary) and left-sided (i.e. mitral and aortic) murmurs can be distinguished based on how breathing affects the amplitude of the murmur. Right-sided murmurs are louder on inspiration, and left-sided murmurs are louder on expiration.

The red cheeks described is a feature of mitral stenosis called malar flush, which is caused by vasodilation of the vascular beds in the cheeks. Other examination findings of mitral stenosis include an irregularly irregular pulse (mitral stenosis can cause AF), a parasternal heave and a loud S1. Rheumatic heart disease is the most common cause of mitral stenosis.

20. A

Epigastric pain that gets worse a few hours after eating is consistent with a duodenal ulcer (as opposed to gastric ulcers which cause pain whilst eating). In addition, long-term use of NSAIDs is a major risk factor for peptic ulcers. Duodenal ulcers are four times more common than gastric ulcers. Other risk factors include chronic use of steroids, aspirin or bisphosphonates, *Helicobacter pylori* infection and alcohol abuse.

H. pylori is the most significant risk factor and should be investigated whenever there is any suspicion of peptic ulcer disease (PUD). There are four ways in which *H. pylori* can be detected: (1) Urea breath test: the patient swallows urea labelled with radioactive carbon-14. If CO_2, containing the labelled carbon, is detected in the patient's breath 10–30 mins later, it suggests that the urea has been cleaved by urease produced by *H. pylori*. (2) Blood antibody test. (3) Stool antigen test. (4) Rapid urease test/Campylobacter-like organism (CLO) test: A biopsy of stomach mucosa is put into a medium containing urea and an indicator. The urease produced by *H. pylori* hydrolyses urea to ammonia, which changes the pH of the medium and makes the indicator change colour. The most appropriate management of *H. pylori*-negative PUD would be stopping NSAIDs and starting omeprazole. Triple therapy is the mainstay of treatment for *H. pylori*-positive PUD and consists of a PPI and two antibiotics.

21. D

Pulmonary fibrosis is an inflammatory condition resulting in fibrosis of the lung parenchyma. The disease falls under the umbrella term of 'interstitial lung disease'. Pulmonary fibrosis causes a chronic dry cough, shortness of breath on exertion and, sometimes, weight loss. Classic examination findings include clubbing and fine inspiratory crackles (usually affecting both lower zones). There are many causes of pulmonary fibrosis including exposure to occupational toxins (e.g. asbestos), systemic inflammatory conditions (e.g. rheumatoid arthritis) and certain medications (e.g. methotrexate). This patient's history of rheumatoid arthritis suggests that the pulmonary fibrosis may be a complication of the disease itself, and/or a complication of its treatment (with methotrexate).

COPD typically causes a productive cough and worsening shortness of breath in patients with an extensive smoking history. Lung cancer usually presents with haemoptysis and is likely to reveal bronchial breathing in a discrete lung zone, as opposed to bilateral fine inspiratory crackles. Bronchiectasis is most often associated with haemoptysis and a cough productive of copious volumes of purulent sputum. TB patients are likely to have a recent history of visiting a TB-endemic region and the disease usually affects the upper lung zones.

Pay attention to every part of the SBA, everything is there for a reason — in this question, you should not discard the history of rheumatoid arthritis as irrelevant additional information.

22. B

This patient is experiencing symptoms of hyperthyroidism (palpitations, sweating and diarrhoea) on a background of a flu-like illness. These symptoms, along with the examination findings of a warm and tender thyroid gland, are indicative of de Quervain's thyroiditis (also known as viral thyroiditis). This condition is caused by viral infection of the thyroid gland, which destroys thyroid follicular cells and halts thyroxine production. Initially, hyperthyroid symptoms are experienced because the destruction of the thyroid gland leads to the release of stored thyroid hormone. After a few weeks, the stored thyroid hormone will run out and the lack of production of new thyroxine by the damaged thyroid gland will result in a phase of hypothyroid symptoms. After a few more weeks, the thyroid gland will recover and the patient will become euthyroid again. Initially, the damaged thyroid follicular cells do not take up any iodine and hence the thyroid gland does not show up on a thyroid uptake scan.

Diffuse uptake throughout an enlarged gland is seen in Graves' disease. A multinodular gland with a single hot nodule is seen in toxic multinodular goitre (also known as Plummer's disease). Diffuse uptake with a single cold nodule may be seen in thyroid cancer.

23. B

A firm, smooth, mobile breast lump without axillary lymphadenopathy, skin changes or nipple discharge in a young woman is more likely to be a fibroadenoma than breast cancer. However, to confidently exclude breast cancer, breast lumps should undergo triple assessment: clinical examination, radiological examination and fine needle aspiration (FNA) or core biopsy. Women under the age of 35 years have very dense breast tissue, meaning that it is difficult to visualise tumours on a mammogram because their normal breast tissue, like tumours, will be radiolucent. Therefore, ultrasound scans are used for the radiological assessment of young women with breast lumps. An FNA may be performed to confirm a diagnosis of fibroadenoma. Most fibroadenomas either stay the same or regress, however, if it is large or causing discomfort to the patient it can be surgically excised. Women over the age of 35 years should be imaged using a two-view mammogram.

24. A

Any patient presenting with acute neurological symptoms (e.g. weakness, slurring of speech, facial droop, amaurosis fugax) that resolve completely within 24 hrs should be given 300 mg aspirin immediately, and assessed urgently within 24 hrs. Patients with confirmed TIAs should then continue antiplatelet medication (aspirin or clopidogrel) and be given medications for secondary prevention (antihypertensives and statins).

A CT head scan is an essential first step in patients presenting with a suspected stroke, to distinguish ischaemic from haemorrhagic. Thrombolysis can be considered in patients with confirmed ischaemic strokes presenting within 4.5 hrs of the onset of symptoms. ECG and carotid Doppler scans are useful when investigating the source of the embolus that caused the TIA. Carotid endarterectomy is considered in patients with >70% stenosis at the origin of the internal carotid artery.

25. D

This child is presenting with the triad of signs and symptoms of Henoch–Schönlein purpura (HSP): arthritis, abdominal pain and a purpuric rash (usually on the buttocks and lower legs). HSP is a form of IgA nephropathy in which immune complexes are deposited in the skin, mucous membranes, joints and organs. HSP mainly occurs in children under the age of 10 years and tends to occur after a respiratory tract infection. Kidney involvement occurs in approximately 40% of cases, presenting with haematuria, proteinuria, hypertension and oedema.

26. B

There are many causes of left iliac fossa pain including diverticulitis, constipation, irritable bowel syndrome, ulcerative colitis (UC), colorectal cancer and gynaecological causes (e.g. pelvic inflammatory disease). Of these, diverticulitis, UC and colorectal cancer are known to cause rectal bleeding. Colorectal cancer tends to be associated with weight loss and UC tends to present in younger patients. Angiodysplasia does cause rectal bleeding, but it is normally painless. Therefore, diverticulitis is the most likely diagnosis as it tends to present between the age of 50 and 70 years. Diverticulae are outpouchings of the mucosa and submucosa that have herniated through the muscularis. Low-fibre diets and constipation are risk factors for the development of diverticulae. They most commonly occur in the sigmoid and descending colon, particularly at the sites of nutrient artery penetration (hence, the rectal bleeding). The terminology can be confusing:

- **Diverticulosis:** the presence of diverticulae.
- **Diverticular disease:** symptomatic diverticulosis (e.g. intermittent lower abdominal pain, bloating, episodes of constipation followed by diarrhoea and rectal bleeding).
- **Diverticulitis:** acute infection and inflammation of the diverticulae, presenting with fever, malaise, nausea and constant left iliac fossa pain.

27. A

Organisms and diseases:

Bordatella pertussis — whooping cough
Treponema pallidum — syphilis
Cryptosporidium — diarrhoeal illness in immunocompromised
    patients
Mycoplasma pneumoniae — atypical pneumonia
Yersinia pestis — the plague

28. B

JVP waveforms are quite difficult to see and interpret, however, they do tend to come up in SBAs. The waveforms correspond with different parts of the cardiac cycle as follows:

> **A wave** = atrial contraction causing some blood to flow back up the superior vena cava
> **C wave** = ventricular contraction causes the tricuspid valve to bulge into the right atrium resulting in a pressure wave passing up the superior vena cava
> **X descent** = atrial relaxation and filling
> **V wave** = caused by increased venous return to the right atrium occurring in late systole
> **Y descent** = flow of blood from the right atrium into the right ventricle through an open tricuspid valve.

Cannon A waves occur when the atria and ventricles contract simultaneously. This results in the right atrium contracting against a closed tricuspid valve and causing a column of blood to shoot up the superior vena cava into the jugular vein. This is most commonly caused by complete heart block.

Large V waves are seen in tricuspid regurgitation. Ventricular contraction causes blood to surge through an incompetent tricuspid valve, through the right atrium and into the jugular vein. Kussmaul sign is a paradoxical rise in JVP on inspiration caused by conditions that impair ventricular filling (e.g. constrictive pericarditis). Raised JVP with absent pulsation occurs in superior vena cava obstruction. Slow Y descent is associated with tricuspid stenosis.

29. A

Ankylosing spondylitis is a seronegative inflammatory arthropathy that mainly affects the axial skeleton and large joints. It is described as 'seronegative' because it shows no significant level of serum antibodies. It is strongly associated with the presence of the HLA-B27 allele. It is more common in males and typically presents with lower back and sacroiliac pain that is worst in the morning and better with activity. It also causes a reduced range of spinal motion. It is diagnosed based on history and examination findings. Schober's test will reveal reduced spinal flexion. Sacroiliitis is an early feature of ankylosing spondylitis, and may be visualised in a plain X-ray of the pelvis.

Lumbar disc herniation is more likely to cause acute back pain with shooting pains in the lower limbs. The location of pain depends on the nerves affected. The straight leg raise is a clinical test that elicits pain in patients with lumbar disc herniation. Osteoarthritis causes joint pain and stiffness that gets worse with joint use. It mainly affects large weight bearing joints, such as the knees, and causes bony swellings along the margins of the small joints in the hands (Heberden's and Bouchard's nodes). A muscle strain is likely to cause pain that is worse with activity. A vertebral fracture would cause sudden-onset back pain with limited spinal mobility.

30. D

The percussion note will be dull (sometimes described as 'stony dull') because of the underlying fluid within the pleura. Vocal resonance and breath sounds will be reduced because sound conducts poorly through fluid.

Percussion note is described as 'resonant' over normal lung tissue, and 'hyper-resonant' over a pneumothorax or a hyperinflated lung (e.g. in COPD). Vocal resonance is increased when the sound travels through an area of con**solid**ation (e.g. tumour, pneumonia) because sound conducts better through **solid**s. Vesicular breath sounds are the normal breath sounds that are heard over areas of normal lung tissue. Bronchial breath sounds are normal when heard over the trachea, however, the presence of bronchial breathing when auscultating other areas of the lungs suggests that there is consolidation in between the surface of the stethoscope and the bronchi (because the sound of air moving through the bronchus (i.e. bronchial breath sounds) conducts via a solid mass to the stethoscope).

Paper 4

Questions

1. A 34-year-old woman is complaining of a drooping eyelid that has been affecting her vision. She has also been suffering from fatigue over the past 3 months, which has impacted on her job as a yoga instructor. She feels relatively fine in the morning, however, she feels very weak towards the end of the day and struggles to complete her evening sessions. What is the most likely diagnosis?

   A Polymyalgia rheumatic
   B Anaemia
   C Myasthenia gravis
   D Lambert-Eaton syndrome
   E Horner's syndrome

2. A 19-year-old asthmatic visits his GP because he is having to use his salbutamol inhaler more than 3 times per week. What is the next step in the management of this patient's asthma?

   A Add oral prednisolone
   B Reassure and send home
   C Increase the dose of inhaled salbutamol
   D Add inhaled salmeterol
   E Add inhaled low-dose beclomethasone

3. A 71-year-old owner of a dye factory presents to his GP having experienced 3 episodes of blood in his urine over the past week. When asked to elaborate, he says that his urine is bright red, however, he experiences no pain when passing urine and has not experienced any trauma to his genitals recently. Otherwise, he has generally been quite healthy although he has noticed that his clothes have become quite loose-fitting despite not having changed his diet or exercised. What is the most likely diagnosis?

    A Pyelonephritis
    B Glomerulonephritis
    C Bladder cancer
    D Prostate cancer
    E Ureteric stone

4. A 44-year-old woman presents with a 7-month history of heartburn, an acidic taste in the back of her mouth and painful swallowing. The GP suspects gastro-oesophageal reflux that is aggravated by a medication that she is taking for a heart condition. Which of the following options could cause or worsen gastro-oesophageal reflux?

    A Beta-blockers
    B ACE inhibitors
    C Nitrates
    D Diuretics
    E Angiotensin receptor blockers

5. A 27-year-old man presents with palpitations and light-headedness. An ECG shows features consistent with a supraventricular tachycardia. Adenosine is administered and the SVT is terminated. A repeat ECG shows a short PR interval and a QRS complex with a slurred upstroke. What is the diagnosis?

    A Brugada syndrome
    B LBBB
    C Romano–Ward syndrome
    D Wolff–Parkinson–White syndrome
    E Complete heart block

6. An 18-year-old man visits his GP complaining of an itchy scalp and nose. He admits that he has been feeling quite self-conscious since a friend pointed out that he has dandruff. On examination, there are patchy erythematous plaques along his scalp covered with yellow scales and white flakes of dead skin in his hair. Similar lesions are also found in the nasolabial folds. Which type of eczema is this likely to be?

    A Nummular
    B Seborrhoeic
    C Contact
    D Atopic
    E Pompholyx

7. Which of the following options fits the criteria for giving long-term oxygen therapy in COPD?

    A PaO_2 7.3–10 kPa despite maximal treatment
    B PaO_2 7.3–10 kPa and pulmonary hypertension
    C PaO_2 < 7.3 kPa despite maximal treatment
    D $PaCO_2$ > 6 kPa despite maximal treatment
    E $PaCO_2$ > 8 kPa despite maximal treatment

8. A 71-year-old female, with a history of atrial fibrillation, presents to A&E with severe, diffuse abdominal pain. Her blood pressure is 84/60 mm Hg and her pulse is irregularly irregular with a rate of 130 bpm. Abdominal examination is normal. An abdominal X-ray is performed. Which of these radiological features is most likely to be seen?

    A Rigler's sign
    B Pneumoperitoneum
    C Toxic megacolon
    D Gasless abdomen
    E Coffee bean sign

9. Which of the following results would you expect to see in a patient with toxic multinodular goitre?

   A High TSH, High TRH & High T3/T4
   B Low TSH, Low TRH & High T3/T4
   C Low TSH, High TRH & High T3/T4
   D High TSH, Low TRH & High T3/T4
   E High TSH, High TRH & Low T3/T4

10. A 68-year-old man has suddenly developed an extremely painful left leg. On examination, his left leg is pale, cold and his dorsalis pedis and posterior tibial pulses are impalpable. His radial pulse is 120 bpm and has an irregularly irregular rhythm. What is the first step in the management of this patient?

   A Duplex ultrasound scan of the lower limb vessels
   B Oral aspirin
   C IV heparin
   D Measure Ankle-Brachial Pressure Index (ABPI)
   E DC cardioversion

11. A 22-year-old man presents with a headache, neck stiffness and photophobia. A diagnosis of viral meningitis is suspected. Once raised ICP is excluded, a lumbar puncture is performed. Which set of results would be consistent with viral meningitis?

   A Cloudy CSF, high neutrophils, high protein and low glucose
   B High lymphocytes, high protein and normal glucose
   C High lymphocytes, low protein and normal glucose
   D High neutrophils, high protein and high glucose
   E Fibrinous CSF, high lymphocytes, high protein and low glucose

12. Which of the following is not a clinical feature of anaemia?

    A Conjunctival pallor
    B Glossitis
    C Angular stomatitis
    D Ruddy/Red complexion
    E Shortness of breath

13. A 39-year-old female presents at her GP practice having coughed up blood last night. This has happened on two previous occasions. She has no significant past medical history although she does experience regular nosebleeds. Blood tests reveal a high ESR and urinalysis reveals proteinuria and haematuria. The presence of which antibody would support the most likely diagnosis?

    A Anti-GBM antibody
    B pANCA
    C cANCA
    D Anti-liver/kidney microsomal antibody
    E Anti-smooth muscle antibody

14. Which of the following is not part of the criteria for diagnosing sepsis?

    A Heart rate > 90 bpm
    B Respiratory rate > 20 breaths per minute
    C Temperature > 38°C
    D White cell count < 4 × 10^9/L
    E Blood pressure < 90/60 mm Hg

15. A 72-year-old patient with severe COPD has recently experienced worsening dyspnoea despite maximal treatment. On examination, he is cyanotic with a raised JVP and ankle oedema. Palpation reveals hepatomegaly. What is the most likely diagnosis?

    A Left ventricular failure
    B Congestive cardiac failure
    C Cor pulmonale
    D Pulmonary hypertension
    E Restrictive cardiomyopathy

16. A 32-year-old man with psoriasis presents to his GP with deformed hands that have been affecting his ability to do his daily tasks. It has gradually got worse over several years. On closer inspection, his fingers are badly deformed and appear to be telescoped. What is the most likely diagnosis?

    A Rheumatoid arthritis
    B Arthritis mutilans
    C Psoriatic spondylopathy
    D Osteoarthritis
    E Distal interphalangeal joint disease

17. A 21-year-old woman has fainted four times in the past 3 months. She becomes sweaty and nauseous before she faints and is usually unconscious for a few seconds. Her friends have told her that she looks abnormally pale before she collapses. She doesn't know if she jerks whilst unconscious, but has not lost control of her bladder or bitten her tongue. When she regains consciousness, she feels slightly dizzy but does not feel confused. What is the most likely cause of her fainting?

    A Hypoglycaemia
    B Epileptic seizure
    C Vasovagal syncope
    D Arrhythmia
    E Hypertrophic obstructive cardiomyopathy

18. A 50-year-old taxi driver attends a GP appointment because he has recently been 'bumping into things' quite regularly and has had to take a break from work over fears about his vision. He struggles to see anything in the left half of his visual field. Examination reveals a left homonymous hemianopia. In which part of the visual pathway is the lesion likely to be located?

    A Optic chiasm
    B Left optic tract
    C Left optic radiation
    D Right optic nerve
    E Right optic tract

19. A 75-year-old woman has had a 3-week history of lower abdominal discomfort and bloating. She is embarrassed to admit that she has recently started wearing adult diapers because she has been soiling her underwear. Her stools are usually very watery and drip into the pan. She has not lost any weight or noticed any blood in the stool. She claims to have a balanced, healthy diet. She has taken codeine every day for the past 4 months since she suffered a hip fracture. On examination, her abdomen is mildly distended and a solid mass is palpated in the left iliac fossa. On digital rectal examination, her underwear is soiled and liquid stool is seen on withdrawal of the finger. What is the most likely diagnosis?

    A Rectal carcinoma
    B Faecal impaction
    C Inguinal hernia
    D Ischaemic colitis
    E Rectocoele

20. A 24-year-old female presents to her GP complaining that her periods have become extremely irregular. She normally has 26–29 day cycles, but in the past 6 months her periods have been much less frequent. On closer inspection, she appears to have an abnormally large amount of facial hair for a young female and she is also suffering from acne, which, she claims, she never had as a teenager. She has gained weight over the past few months, which, alongside the acne and facial hair growth, has made her feel depressed. What is the most likely diagnosis?

    A Hypothyroidism
    B Turner's syndrome
    C Polycystic ovarian syndrome
    D Pregnancy
    E Panhypopituitarism

21. Which of the following is a respiratory cause of asterixis?

    A Hypoxia
    B Carbon dioxide retention
    C Salbutamol side-effect
    D Secondary polycythaemia
    E Bronchiectasis

22. A 23-year-old student has arranged an appointment with his GP to discuss his 'incredibly itchy' eyes. Yesterday morning he noticed that his left eye became quite red and itchy, and started watering. A few hours later, his right eye also started to display the same symptoms. On closer inspection, both eyes show conjunctival injection and watering. A yellow crust is seen across the margins of the eyelids. What is the most likely diagnosis?

    A Hypopyon
    B Hyphaema
    C Bacterial conjunctivitis
    D Viral conjunctivitis
    E Uveitis

23. A 53-year-old man visits his GP to discuss a swollen scrotum that has caused him some discomfort and much embarrassment since he first noticed it 3 weeks ago. The swelling has grown gradually and, although it is uncomfortable, it is not painful. He reports no difficulties with passing urine. On examination, his left hemiscrotum is considerably enlarged, fluctuant and non-tender. It is possible to get above the swelling, however, the left testicle cannot be distinguished. When a pen torch is shone on the swelling, it illuminates brightly. What is the most likely diagnosis?

    A Varicocoele
    B Hydrocoele
    C Testicular tumour
    D Epididymal cyst
    E Indirect inguinal hernia

24. A 52-year-old man has been experiencing some chest pain and short-ness of breath, which is worse when lying down. He has also col-lapsed 3 times in the past couple of months. His father died of a heart condition when he was 58 years old, although he cannot recall the details of the condition. On examination, a jerky carotid pulse is pal-pated and a crescendo-decrescendo murmur is heard over the carotid artery. What is the most likely diagnosis?

    A Aortic stenosis
    B Hypertrophic obstructive cardiomyopathy
    C Left heart failure
    D Mitral regurgitation
    E Constrictive pericarditis

25. A 48-year-old man has been in hospital for 2 days receiving treatment for pneumonia. He has a past medical history of acute pancreatitis, which occurred 3 years ago. He has a long history of alcohol abuse. In the last hour, he has started sweating excessively, complains of palpitations and appears very anxious. He is clearly agitated and begins shouting at the nurses to 'get these creatures off me!' What is the most appropriate treatment?

    A Diazepam
    B Phenobarbital
    C Loperamide
    D Chlordiazepoxide
    E Risperidone

26. A 56-year-old man has recently registered at a new GP practice. As part of the registration process, he has been asked to undergo some routine blood tests. FBC reveals the following results:

    Hb: 106 g/L (130–180)
    WBC: 95×10^9 /L (4–11)
    Platelets: 86×10^9/L (150–400)
    Lymphocytes: 85×10^9 (1.5–4.5)

A diagnosis of chronic lymphocytic leukaemia is suspected. Which of the following features are you most likely to see on his blood film?

A Smear cells
B Atypical lymphocytes
C Auer rods
D Reed–Sternberg cells
E Schistocytes

27. A 21-year-old university student presents with a 1-week history of sore throat, fever and malaise. On examination, there is cervical lymphadenopathy, splenomegaly and inflamed tonsils. The GP diagnoses the patient with bacterial tonsillitis and prescribes ampicillin. The patient comes back 2-days later with a widespread maculopapular rash. What is the underlying diagnosis?

A Penicillin allergy
B Erythema multiforme
C Stevens–Johnson syndrome
D Infectious mononucleosis
E Idiopathic thrombocytopaenic purpura

28. A 47-year-old man presents to his GP having experienced a few episodes of haemoptysis over the past month. He returned from a holiday to Bangladesh 6 weeks ago. On direct questioning, he admits to losing approximately 5 kg in weight over the past month and he has had to replace his bed sheets more frequently because they are often drenched with sweat when he wakes up in the morning. A chest X-ray reveals an area of consolidation in the right upper zone. Sputum microscopy using Ziehl–Neelsen stain reveals acid-fast bacilli. What is the most appropriate treatment option?

A Rifampicin and isoniazid for 6 months; ethambutol and pyrazinamide for the first 2 months
B Ethambutol and pyrazinamide for 6 months; rifampicin and isoniazid for the first 2 months

C Rifampicin and isoniazid for 6 months; ethambutol and pyrazinamide for the first 4 months

D Rifampicin and pyrazinamide for 6 months; ethambutol and isoniazid for the first 2 months

E Rifampicin, pyrazinamide, ethambutol and isoniazid for 6 months

29. A 23-year-old university student is brought to A&E at 2 am by his friends. He is clearly inebriated and struggles to maintain conversation. His friends explain that he had been celebrating the recent election results at a bar when he began to vomit. He vomited several times and splashes of 'bright red' blood was seen the last two times that he vomited. What is the most likely diagnosis?

   A Peptic ulcer disease
   B Boerhaave syndrome
   C Mallory–Weiss syndrome
   D Gastritis
   E Osler–Weber–Rendu syndrome

30. A 65-year-old man is brought in to A&E by his wife. She says that he has been very confused over the last few days and has fallen over several times. She adds that her husband has wet the bed twice over the last 2 days — this has never happened before. What is the most likely diagnosis?

   A Alzheimer's disease
   B Obstructive hydrocephalus
   C UTI
   D Subdural haematoma
   E Normal pressure hydrocephalus

Answers

1. C

Myasthenia gravis is an autoimmune disease of the neuromuscular junctions characterised by the destruction of nicotinic acetylcholine receptors leading to weakness in various muscle groups across the body. Eye signs, such as ptosis and fatigue of extra-ocular muscles, are early features of myasthenia gravis. The disease can also affect bulbar muscles (those supplied by cranial nerves 9–12), leading to difficulty in swallowing and chewing. Generalised weakness affecting multiple muscle groups is also common. Myasthenia gravis is characterised by fatigue that gets worse with activity — patients often complain about severe fatigue towards the end of the day.

Lambert-Eaton syndrome is a paraneoplastic disease caused by the destruction of pre-synaptic calcium channels, which presents very similarly to myasthenia gravis. However, fatigue, in Lambert-Eaton syndrome, improves with activity. Polymyalgia rheumatica is an inflammatory condition, which causes pain and stiffness (*without* weakness) of the shoulder and pelvic girdle that is typically worst in the morning. Anaemia causes gradual onset fatigue; however, it would not cause ptosis. Horner's syndrome is caused by disruption of the sympathetic nervous supply to the head and neck. Its main features are ptosis, miosis and anhidrosis. Causes include apical lung tumours, strokes, and carotid artery dissection.

2. E

Asthma management is an important topic that often comes up in OSCEs and SBAs. The British Thoracic Society (BTS) guidelines for asthma management are simplified below:

STEP 1: Inhaled short-acting beta agonist (e.g. salbutamol)
STEP 2: Inhaled corticosteroid (e.g. beclomethasone)
STEP 3: Inhaled long-acting beta agonist (e.g. salmeterol) + consider increasing dose of inhaled corticosteroid
STEP 4: Consider trials of theophylline, oral beta agonists, oral leukotriene receptor antagonists (Montelukast therapy)
STEP 5: Oral corticosteroids

This patient is currently on Step 1, however, he is having to use his salbutamol inhaler more than three times per week. This is an indication that the patient's asthma management needs to be escalated. The next step would be adding an inhaled corticosteroid (e.g. inhaled low-dose beclomethasone).

3. C

The main symptom of bladder cancer is painless macroscopic haematuria. Some patients may experience some storage symptoms such as frequency, urgency and nocturia but this is very variable. Patients are also likely to experience systemic symptoms of malignancy, such as weight loss. Bladder cancer can either be a transitional cell carcinoma (most common) or a squamous cell carcinoma. Bladder cancer is strongly associated with exposure to dye-stuffs — this patient's history as the owner of a dye factory suggests that he is at risk. Suspected bladder cancer is investigated using cystoscopy and biopsy.

Pyelonephritis will cause haematuria and symptoms of infection (e.g. high fever). Glomerulonephritis usually causes microscopic haematuria. Prostate cancer is likely to cause very pronounced voiding symptoms (e.g. hesitancy, poor stream, terminal dribbling). A ureteric stone will cause microscopic haematuria and is likely to present as an emergency with the patient suffering from excruciating, colicky 'loin to groin' pain.

4. C

This patient is presenting with typical features of GORD. Inflammation of the oesophagus, due to the reflux of gastric acid, will cause episodic heartburn. There are several medications that can exacerbate symptoms of reflux including drugs that damage the mucosa (e.g. NSAIDs, aspirin, steroids and bisphosphonates) and drugs that affect oesophageal motility (e.g. TCAs, nitrates and anticholinergics). Nitrates are smooth muscle relaxants which reduce the contraction of the lower oesophageal sphincter, thus increasing the risk of acid reflux. They are used to treat angina by causing coronary artery vasodilation and improving myocardial perfusion. GORD is managed with lifestyle interventions such as stopping smoking, avoiding spicy food, losing weight, having small, regular meals and avoiding eating before bed. Patients are usually started on a once daily PPI and patients who do not respond should be offered twice daily PPIs.

5. D

'Supraventricular tachycardia' technically means any tachycardia that originates above the ventricles, however, the term tends to, more specifically, refer to atrioventricular re-entry tachycardia (AVRT) and atrioventricular nodal re-entry tachycardia (AVNRT). AVRT occurs when a re-entry circuit is established between the atria and the ventricles via an accessory pathway known as the bundle of Kent. Once an SVT is terminated, depolarisation will still travel down the bundle of Kent and cause 'pre-excitation' of the ventricles, producing a slurred upstroke and a short PR interval on the ECG. The presence of an accessory pathway, pre-excitation of the ventricles and a tendency to develop SVTs is known as Wolff–Parkinson–White syndrome.

Brugada syndrome is a rare but well-known genetic disease associated with sudden death in adults. Left bundle-branch block would produce wide QRS complexes with a 'W' shape in V1 and an 'M' shape in V6. The bundle-branch block ECG features can be remembered using the famous 'WiLLiaM MaRRoW' method. Romano–Ward syndrome is a hereditary condition that causes long QT syndrome and is also associated with sudden death. Complete heart block causes bradycardia, broad QRS complexes and complete dissociation between p waves and QRS complexes.

6. B

Seborrhoeic eczema (also known as seborrhoeic dermatitis) most commonly affects areas rich in sebaceous glands such as the scalp, eyebrows and nasolabial folds. It is thought to be caused by an inflammatory reaction to an overgrowth of *Pityrosporum* yeast and usually begins on the scalp as dandruff. It later progresses to redness and irritation with the development of yellow, greasy scales overlying the inflamed skin. Lesions may spread from the scalp to the forehead, post-auricular skin and posterior part of the neck. Seborrhoeic eczema may also be seen on other parts of the body including the armpits, under the breasts and between the buttocks.

Nummular (discoid) eczema consists of very distinct coin-shaped lesions which are usually seen on the shins, forearms and trunk. Contact eczema is a type IV delayed hypersensitivity reaction to an allergen, for example, soap, nickel, tobacco smoke and paint. It affects the part of the body that has been exposed to the allergen — often the hands. Atopic eczema is the most common type of eczema, forming part of the atopic triad (along with hay fever and asthma). It is most commonly seen in children and usually affects the face and skin folds (e.g. neck, wrists and cubital fossa). Pompholyx eczema consists of fluid-filled blisters restricted to the palms of the hands and soles of the feet.

7. C

The NICE guidelines suggest that long-term oxygen therapy should be considered in the following groups of patients:

- Patients with PaO_2 < 7.3 kPa despite maximal treatment
- Patients with PaO_2 7.3–8.0 kPa and one of: pulmonary hypertension, polycythaemia, peripheral oedema or nocturnal hypoxia
- Terminally ill patients

8. D

This patient is presenting with a triad of features associated with acute mesenteric ischaemia: Severe abdominal pain, normal abdominal examination and shock. This is characterised by vascular compromise of the small bowel due to occlusion of the superior mesenteric artery — it can be classified as acute or chronic. Acute disease occurs due to arterial thrombosis (e.g. due to atherosclerosis) or embolism (e.g. due to emboli from AF). Other causes of acute mesenteric ischaemia include venous thrombosis (in hypercoagulable states) and non-occlusive disease (e.g. hypotension). Chronic mesenteric ischaemia usually occurs due to a combination of a low-flow state, such as heart failure, and atherosclerotic disease. It presents with 'gut claudication' (poorly localised, colicky, postprandial abdominal pain), PR bleeding and weight loss. Patients with suspected mesenteric ischaemia should have an abdominal X-ray. In advanced disease, it may show a gasless abdomen, thickening of the bowel wall and pneumatosis (air within the bowel wall due to necrosis). If the abdominal X-ray is inconclusive, a CT scan should be performed.

Rigler's sign (air present on both sides of the bowel wall, creating the impression of a 'double wall') and pneumoperitoneum (air under the diaphragm) are signs of perforation. Toxic megacolon is a complication of UC characterised by non-obstructive colonic dilatation (>6 cm) and systemic toxicity (e.g. fever, tachycardia, leukocytosis). Coffee bean sign is a radiological feature of sigmoid volvulus, in which the sigmoid colon twists on its mesentery causing a strangulated obstruction.

9. B

Toxic multinodular goitre, also known as Plummer's disease, is when a nodule, within a multinodular thyroid gland, stops responding to TSH-mediated feedback and begins to produce T3/T4 autonomously. This leads to a very high T3/T4. The high levels of circulating thyroid hormone, via a negative feedback loop, reduces the release of TRH (from the hypothalamus) and TSH (from the pituitary gland). This results in: Low TSH, Low TRH & High T3/T4.

10. C

This patient is presenting with acute limb ischaemia — a surgical emergency arising from the sudden cessation of blood flow to a limb. The features of acute limb ischaemia are remembered as 'the 6 Ps': **P**ale, **P**ulseless, **P**ainful, **P**aralysis, **P**araesthesia and **P**erishingly cold. It can be caused by a thrombus *in situ* or by an embolus (e.g. from AF). Patients with suspected acute limb ischemia should immediately receive IV heparin and be referred to the vascular surgery department. Heparinisation should not be delayed by investigations. Definitive treatment options include surgical embolectomy and thrombolysis.

Duplex ultrasound can assess the extent and location of the stenoses. ABPI is a simple test that can indicate the presence of peripheral vascular disease. IV heparin is preferred over oral aspirin to provide anticoagulation in acute limb ischaemia. DC cardioversion may be appropriate to treat this patient's AF, however, it is not the most appropriate first step.

11. B

The most common causes of viral meningitis are enteroviruses (e.g. polio-virus, Coxsackie A) and Herpes viruses (e.g. HSV, VZV, EBV). Like its bacterial counterpart, viral meningitis characteristically presents with a headache, neck stiffness, fever and photophobia. However, symptoms are often less severe and do not progress as quickly. Diagnosis is based on lumbar puncture and CSF analysis. Remember, raised ICP should be excluded before an LP is performed to prevent brainstem herniation. This table lists the key differences in CSF characteristics in meningitis caused by bacteria, viruses and TB:

Diagnosis	Appearance	Predominant cell type	Protein concentration	Glucose concentration
Bacterial	Cloudy/turbis	Neutrophils	High	Low
Viral	Usually clear	Lymphocytes	High	Normal
TB	Fibrinous	Lymphocytes	High	Low

12. D

A ruddy/red complexion is a feature of polycythaemia. Common features of anaemia include conjunctival pallor, shortness of breath, tachycardia and lethargy. Glossitis and angular stomatitis occur in iron, folate and vitamin B12 deficiency anaemia.

13. C

Granulomatosis with polyangiitis (previously known as Wegener's granulomatosis) is a systemic vasculitis that is characterised by a triad of upper and lower respiratory tract involvement (nosebleeds and haem-optysis) and glomerulonephritis (haematuria and proteinuria). A 'saddle nose' is another clinical feature of granulomatosis with polyangiitis, which is sometimes mentioned in SBAs. It is strongly associated with the presence of cytoplasmic anti-neutrophil cytoplasmic antibodies (cANCA).

Anti-GBM antibodies are the hallmark of Goodpasture's syndrome — an autoimmune condition attacking the basement membrane in the kidneys and lungs leading to renal failure and haemoptysis. Nose bleeds are not a feature of Goodpasture's syndrome. Perinuclear anti-neutrophil cytoplasmic antibody (pANCA) is associated with several inflammatory conditions including ulcerative colitis, primary sclerosing cholangitis, microscopic polyangiitis and Churg–Strauss syndrome. Anti-liver/kidney microsomal (anti-LKM) antibodies and anti-smooth muscle antibodies (ASMA) are present in autoimmune hepatitis.

14. E

Systemic inflammatory response syndrome (SIRS) is defined by the following parameters:

- Heart rate > 90 bpm
- Respiratory rate > 20/min or $PaCO_2$ < 4.3 kPa
- Temperature > 38°C or < 36°C
- White cell count < 4×10^9/L or > 12×10^9/L

Sepsis is a spectrum with varying degrees of severity. Septicaemia refers to the presence of an organism within the blood. Sepsis is, in simple terms, the combination of septicaemia and SIRS. Severe sepsis occurs when septic patients begins to show evidence of organ hypoperfusion (e.g. elevated serum lactate). Septic shock is a combination of sepsis and refractory hypotension. This can lead to organ failure and death.

15. C

Cor pulmonale is right heart failure resulting from chronic pulmonary hypertension. Underlying causes include chronic lung diseases (e.g. COPD), pulmonary vascular disease (e.g. PE) and neuromuscular disease (e.g. myasthenia gravis). Symptoms include shortness of breath and fatigue. The signs of cor pulmonale resemble right ventricular failure: cyanosis, raised JVP, hepatomegaly and oedema. A pansystolic murmur (due to tricuspid regurgitation) or a Graham-Steell murmur (due to pulmonary regurgitation) may be heard. Cor pulmonale has a poor prognosis — 50% will die within 5 years.

16. B

This patient has psoriatic arthritis, which is (rather obviously) when someone with psoriasis develops arthritis. There are five main presentations of psoriatic arthritis: distal interphalangeal joint disease, psoriatic spondylopathy (mainly involving the axial skeleton), symmetrical polyarthritis, asymmetrical oligoarthritis and arthritis mutilans ('telescoping' of the digits). Be sure to look up an image of arthritis mutilans — you'll never forget it.

17. C

The most common cause of fainting in young people is vasovagal syncope. This occurs when vagal discharge causes bradycardia and peripheral vasodilation, leading to cerebral hypoperfusion and syncope. Patients usually describe a warning or presyncopal sensation, such as an odd sensation in the stomach, going pale and clammy or feeling dizzy. There is often a precipitating factor such as prolonged standing, pain, extremes of emotion, micturition, straining, coughing and exercise. Vasovagal syncope tends to last for a few seconds and twitching and incontinence rarely occur during these episodes.

This is unlikely to be an epileptic seizure as there was no tongue biting, aura or post-ictal confusion. An arrhythmia is also unlikely as she did not experience any chest pain or palpitations prior to the episode and the event was not triggered by exercise. When answering a syncope question or taking a syncope history, it is important to consider what happened before, during and after the episode. These differences are summarised in the table below:

	Epilepsy	**Vasovagal**	**Arrhythmia**
Before	Aura (Partial seizure) No warning (generalised seizure)	Vagal symptoms (sweating, pallor, nausea) Precipitants (e.g. hot weather)	Chest pain Palpitations No warning
During	Minutes Tongue biting Limb jerking Incontinence	Seconds Rarely twitching and incontinence	Seconds
After	Slow recovery Confusion	Rapid recovery on sitting or lying	Rapid spontaneous recovery

Fainting caused by hypoglycaemia is likely to mention a past medical history of diabetes as well as missed meals or inappropriate insulin administration. Hypoglycaemic symptoms such as sweating and nausea may also be described.

18. E

Light is detected by rods and cones in the retina, which then generate an electrical signal that passes along the optic nerve. The optic nerve contains two main bundles of nerves, one will carry signals from the medial half of the retina (responsible for the temporal half of the visual field) and the other will carry signals from the lateral half of the retina (responsible for the nasal half of the visual field). The two optic nerves will meet at a point called the optic chiasma. At the chiasm, the neurons from the lateral half of the retina will continue to the optic tract on the ipsilateral side. Whereas the neurons from the medial half of the retina will decussate at the chiasm and join the optic tract on the contralateral side. Therefore, the optic tract in the left hemisphere is responsible for the right half of the visual field and the optic tract in the right hemisphere is responsible for the left half of the visual field. The optic tract ends at the lateral geniculate nucleus (LGN) in the thalamus. Optic radiations link the LGN to the visual cortex. The optic radiations have an upper division (passing through the parietal lobe) and a lower division (passing through the temporal lobe). The upper division is responsible for the inferior quadrant of the visual field (e.g. the upper division of the optic radiation in the right hemisphere is responsible for the left inferior quadrant) and the lower division is responsible for the superior quadrant. The primary visual cortex will then integrate the information from these inputs.

Damage to the optic nerve will lead to complete loss of vision in one eye, with intact vision in the other eye. Disruption of the optic chiasm (e.g. by pituitary tumours) mainly affects the neurons from the medial half of the retina, which decussates at the chiasm. This leads to bitemporal hemianopia. The optic tract carries information from one half of the visual field — i.e. right half of the visual field in the left optic tract and vice versa. Disruption of this tract leads to homonymous hemianopia (loss of one half of the visual field). Disruption of the upper and lower divisions of the optic radiations will lead to superior or inferior homonymous quadrantopia.

This patient has left homonymous hemianopia, meaning that his right optic tract has been damaged.

19. B

Lower abdominal pain, bloating, abdominal distension and the presence of a palpable mass in the left iliac fossa is suggestive of constipation. This is supported by her medication history — constipation is a very common side-effect of codeine (and other opioids such as morphine). Faecal impaction in the distal colon can lead to liquid stools leaking through the little space left in the lumen causing, what is known as, over-flow diarrhoea. It can lead to faecal incontinence. There are many causes of constipation including dehydration, lack of dietary fibre, physical inactivity, medication and gastrointestinal diseases (e.g. diverticular disease, IBS).

Ischaemic colitis and rectal carcinoma are likely to cause rectal bleeding. Inguinal hernias tend to present as painless lumps upon straining. They can become incarcerated or strangulated causing an obstruction that leads to constipation, however, this is like to present acutely. A rectocoele is a herniation of the rectum into the vagina due to a tear in the rectovaginal septum. Patients may experience constipation, tenesmus, faecal incontinence and dyspareunia.

20. C

Polycystic ovarian syndrome (PCOS) is characterised by oligomenor-rhoea/amenorrhoea and features of hyperandrogenism. Although the exact cause of PCOS is unknown, the disease has a very strong genetic compo-nent, which follows an autosomal dominant pattern with variable expres-sivity. Presenting symptoms include menstrual irregularities, hirsuitism, male-pattern hair loss and acne. PCOS is the most common cause of infertility in women. Other associations of PCOS include obesity, insulin resistance, type 2 diabetes mellitus and dyslipidaemia. Cushing's syndrome can have a very similar presentation to PCOS.

Turner syndrome is a chromosomal abnormality in which females are born with only one X chromosome. Features include short-stature, low posterior hair line, primary amenorrhoea and webbed neck. Pregnancy does cause weight gain and secondary amenorrhoea but will not cause features of hyperandrogenism. Panhypopituitarism will cause more widespread endocrinopathies, including hypoadrenalism and hypothyroidism.

21. B

Asterixis, sometimes called a 'flapping tremor' or 'liver flap', is a tremor that occurs when the wrist is extended. It signifies an inability to maintain posture due to metabolic encephalopathy. Causes include hepatic encephalopathy, azotaemia due to renal failure, carbon dioxide retention, Wilson's disease and drugs-induced (e.g. phenytoin). Salbutamol may cause a fine tremor in the hands but it will not cause a flapping tremor.

22. C

Conjunctivitis refers to inflammation of the conjunctiva which is usually caused by infection. It typically presents with very itchy, red eyes which feel gritty and have started to water. Initially, the disease may only affect one eye but it will usually become bilateral. The cornea, iris and visual acuity will remain normal. Bacterial conjunctivitis may cause a purulent discharge ('yellow crust') whereas viral conjunctivitis will only make the eyes water.

A hypopyon is a yellow exudate seen in the lower part of the anterior chamber of the eye, associated with corneal ulcers. A hyphaema is a collection of blood in the anterior chamber, usually caused by injury to the eye. Uveitis is inflammation of the uvea, which is a manifestation of many systemic diseases including Crohn's disease, Behçet's disease and granulomatosis with polyangiitis.

23. B

A hydrocoele is an accumulation of fluid within the tunica vaginalis (a serous lining around the testis). It can be idiopathic or it can occur secondary to infection, tumours and trauma. Scrotal swellings can be diagnosed quite methodically based on various clinical findings. Inguinal hernias cause scrotal lumps that you 'cannot get above' as the hernial sac extends all the way up to the superficial inguinal ring, where it emerges from the inguinal canal. A painless lump that can be palpated separate to the testicle is likely to be an epididymal cyst or a varicocoele (abnormal dilation of the pampiniform plexus). In SBAs, varicocoeles are often described as feeling like a 'bag of worms'. A painless mass that cannot be distinguished from the testicle (as in this patient) may be a hydrocoele or a testicular tumour. Shining a light onto the swelling is a technique known as transillumination. Fluid-filled masses such as cysts and hydrocoeles will be bright as the light passes through the fluid. This allows cystic swellings to be distinguished from other swellings. Painful and tender swellings are likely to be caused by infection or acute bleeds. This patient has a painless scrotal swelling that you can get above but is indistinguishable from the testicle. Furthermore, it is fluctuant and transilluminates meaning that this is most likely to be a hydrocoele.

24. B

Cardiomyopathy is a primary disease of the myocardium, which has three main types: dilated, restrictive and hypertrophic obstructive. Dilated cardiomyopathy can be inherited, but it is also associated with alcohol abuse, post-viral myocarditis and thyrotoxicosis. In restrictive cardiomyopathy, the stiff ventricles are unable to relax and adequately fill with blood. Causes include amyloidosis, sarcoidosis and haemochromatosis. Hypertrophic obstructive cardiomyopathy (HOCM) has a strong genetic component with roughly 50% of cases being inherited in an autosomal dominant fashion. HOCM can cause sudden death in adults, so it is important to enquire about a family history of sudden death (typically below the age of 65 years). Cardiomyopathy, in general, can present with chest pain, syncope and symptoms of heart failure. HOCM can be distinguished from other forms of cardiomyopathy because it has several specific clinical findings on examination: jerky carotid pulse, ejection systolic murmur and a double apex beat. As this patient has a family history of sudden death and demonstrates some of these specific signs, HOCM is the most likely diagnosis. This can be confirmed using echocardiography — which shows thickened ventricular walls. Cardiac catheterization is sometimes used to measure the pressures in the left ventricle and aorta.

25. D

The symptoms of alcohol withdrawal are very varied. Mild symptoms include restlessness, tremor, sweating and palpitations. If severe, patients will experience hallucinations (often of insects crawling on them — a feeling known as formication) and seizures. Delirium tremens is an acute confusional state seen in chronic alcoholics undergoing withdrawal — it is characterised by anxiety, tremor, sweating, and hallucinations. It can be fatal. Chlordiazepoxide is a benzodiazepine that reduces the effects of alcohol withdrawal and is the best medication to use in this patient. Pabrinex is a mixture of soluble vitamins (including thiamine), which is also given to patients with a history of alcoholism. This prevents the development of Wernicke–Korsakoff syndrome.

Diazepam is another benzodiazepine that can be used to reduce the symptoms of alcohol withdrawal, however, chlordiazepoxide is more commonly used. Phenobarbital is a barbiturate that is sometimes used in the treatment of epilepsy. Loperamide is a weak opioid used as an antidiarrhoeal. Risperidone is an antipsychotic used in the treatment of schizophrenia and bipolar disorder.

26. A

This patient has been diagnosed with chronic lymphocytic leukaemia (CLL) — a malignant proliferation of functionally inept monoclonal lymphocytes. CLL is often asymptomatic, but patients may present with non-specific symptoms (e.g. lethargy, malaise) and symptoms of bone marrow failure (e.g. anaemia, recurrent infections, easy bruising or bleeding). A full blood count will reveal high lymphocytes, low platelets and low haemoglobin. All the leukaemias and lymphomas can get quite confusing because they have similar symptoms, however, each of them has one or two specific associations that are commonly seen in SBAs:

Acute Myeloid Leukaemia (AML)	Auer rods
	Sudan black stain
Acute Lymphoblastic Leukaemia (ALL)	Occurs in children
Chronic Myeloid Leukaemia (CML)	Philadelphia Chromosome (translocation between Chr 9 and 22)
	Massive splenomegaly
Chronic Lymphocytic Leukaemia (CLL)	Smear/Smudge cells
	Warm agglutinins (AIHA)
Hodgkin's Lymphoma	Painful lymph nodes after alcohol ingestion
	Reed-Sternberg cells
	B symptoms (fever, weight loss, night sweats)
Non-Hodgkin's Lymphoma	Painless, enlarging cervical lymph nodes
	B symptoms (fever, weight loss, night sweats)
Myelodysplasia	Ringed sideroblasts
	No splenomgealy
Myelofibrosis	*Massive* splenomegaly
	Dry tap (failure of bone marrow aspirate)
	Dacrocytes (tear drop cells)
	Associated with polycythaemia rubra vera

27. D

The non-specific flu-like symptoms (fever, malaise, sore throat) along with cervical lymphadenopathy and splenomegaly is typical of infectious mononucleosis (also known as glandular fever). Ampicillin and amoxicillin should *not* be given to patients with suspected infectious mononucleosis because it causes a widespread maculopapular rash in nearly all of these patients.

Penicillin allergy is more likely to present with the classic features of an allergic reaction (e.g. wheeze, rash, swelling). Erythema multiforme is a hypersensitivity reaction of the skin that causes target-shaped red lesions.

Stevens–Johnson syndrome is a severe form of erythema multiforme resulting in bullous lesions and necrotic ulcers. It is most commonly associated with the use of anti-epileptic drugs (e.g. lamotrigine). Idiopathic thrombocytopaenic purpura (ITP) is characterised by immune-mediated destruction of platelets leading to a purpuric rash, easy bruising and bleeding. Acute ITP often occurs after viral infections in children.

28. A

Tuberculosis treatment is a very simple SBA topic, however, the wording of the question can be confusing. First and foremost, this is a very typical SBA presentation of TB — an individual presenting with haemoptysis, weight loss and night sweats having recently visited a country known to have TB (e.g. Bangladesh). Lung cancer would be an appropriate differential, however, the X-ray and microbiology findings confirm a diagnosis of TB. The treatment of TB is as follows — make sure you are VERY clear about it:

All four drugs are started *at the same time*

Rifampicin and **I**soniazid — 6 months

Pyrazinamide and **E**thambutol — 2 months

These drugs can be remembered using the mnemonic: **RIPE**

N.B. Pyridoxine (vitamin B6) is given alongside TB treatment because isoniazid leads to vitamin B6 deficiency, which causes peripheral neuropathy.

29. C

Mallory–Weiss syndrome is a tear in the oesophageal mucosa caused by forceful vomiting or retching. Severe vomiting after an alcohol binge is a well-documented cause of Mallory–Weiss syndrome, and it often crops up in SBAs. Patients may present complaining that they are 'vomiting blood', however, Mallory–Weiss tears usually occur after a period of vomiting stomach contents without blood. So, it is important to ask the patient to clarify whether the vomit was normal (i.e. not blood-stained) to begin with and then became blood-stained later on. Mallory–Weiss tears usually heal by themselves. Boerhaave syndrome is a related, but much more serious, condition in which there is a full thickness tear in the oesophagus.

Peptic ulcer disease can cause haematemesis but the patient is also likely to report a change in the stools (digestion of blood leads to black, tarry stools — 'melaena') and epigastric pain. Gastritis is also likely to cause epigastric pain and it may also cause bloating and belching. Osler–Weber–Rendu syndrome, also known as hereditary haemorrhagic telangiectasia, is an autosomal dominant condition that leads to the formation of abnormal blood vessels (telangiectases) in the skin and mucous membranes. Telangiectases can be found along the GI tract and are prone to bleeding, which can manifest as haematemesis or rectal bleeding.

30. E

This patient is presenting with a triad of symptoms associated with normal pressure hydrocephalus (NPH): confusion/dementia, gait disturbance and urinary incontinence. NPH is characterised by enlargement of the lateral ventricles in response to an accumulation of CSF — the intracranial pressure (ICP) remains normal. It is a subtype of non-obstructive hydrocephalus, usually diagnosed using a CT scan.

Obstructive hydrocephalus can also cause confusion, however, it usually presents with a rapid drop in consciousness (if acute) and signs of raised ICP (e.g. Cushing's triad, headache that worsens when lying down), which are not seen in this patient. Falls, confusion and urinary incontinence are features of Alzheimer's disease, but would be seen in patients with advanced disease rather than in a patient presenting acutely. Subdural haematoma presents with headache and fluctuating consciousness — it typically follows head trauma.

Paper 5

Questions

1. Which of the following is a feature of limited cutaneous systemic sclerosis?

   A Calcinosis
   B Cyanosis
   C Striae
   D Onycholysis
   E Clubbing

2. A 32-year-old basketball player is brought to A&E extremely breathless. He was at basketball training when he suddenly felt himself getting more and more breathless and developed a 'stabbing' pain on the right side of his chest. He has never experienced anything like this before. On examination, he is very tall and thin, and breath sounds are reduced over the right side of his chest. What is the most likely diagnosis?

   A PE
   B Primary pneumothorax
   C Secondary pneumothorax
   D Myocardial infarction
   E Asthma attack

3. A 22-year-old student presents with a severe headache and fever that has lasted 1 day. On examination, he has a stiff neck and a rash across his arms and legs. The junior doctor gently flexes the patient's neck. As he does this, the patient's hips flex. What is the name of this sign?

    A Uhthoff's sign
    B Lhermitte's sign
    C Kernig's sign
    D Brudzinski's sign
    E Tinel's sign

4. A 61-year-old woman visits the GP complaining of 13 kg of weight loss over the past 6 months. On direct questioning, she admits that her faeces are lighter in colour than normal and her urine has become darker. She is jaundiced and a large non-tender mass is palpated in her right upper quadrant. What is the most likely diagnosis?

    A Gallstones
    B Hepatocellular carcinoma
    C Pancreatic cancer
    D Bile duct stricture
    E Cirrhosis

5. A 46-year-old man has been admitted to A&E after experiencing palpitations, which began about 4 hours ago. An ECG is performed, which reveals atrial fibrillation. He has no previous history of ischaemic heart disease. He refuses DC cardioversion. What is the next most appropriate treatment option?

    A Defibrillation
    B Low molecular weight heparin
    C Warfarin
    D Flecainide
    E Digoxin

6. A 4-year-old boy is referred to the paediatric department by his GP after a 3-week history of fatigue, shortness of breath and recurrent chest infections. A thorough examination is performed, which revealed extensive bruising across the child's body, hepatosplenomegaly and cervical lymphadenopathy. Based on the information provided, what is the most likely diagnosis?

   A Acute lymphoblastic leukaemia
   B Acute myeloid leukaemia
   C Chronic lymphocytic leukaemia
   D Chronic lymphoblastic leukaemia
   E Hodgkin's lymphoma

7. A 79-year-old woman is accompanied by her granddaughter to A&E. She has had a productive cough and a fever for the past 4 days. On examination, she has an AMTS of 5/10, respiratory rate of 31/min and blood pressure of 92/66 mm Hg. Her urea is 3 mmol/L (2.5–6.7). A CXR reveals an area of consolidation in the right middle lobe. Community-acquired pneumonia is suspected. What is her CURB-65 score?

   A There is not enough information to tell
   B 2
   C 3
   D 4
   E 5

8. A 28-year-old man has experienced several episodes of sweating, palpitations and anxiety over the past 6 months. He has a past medical history of thyroid cancer (aged 19) which was treated with total thyroidectomy. What is the most appropriate investigation?

   A Serum 17-hydroxyprogesterone levels
   B 24-hr urine 5-hydroxyindoleacetic acid levels
   C 24-hr urine vanillylmendelic acid
   D Plasma adrenaline concentration
   E Thyroid uptake scan

9. Which of the following triads best describes Horner's syndrome?

    A Ptosis, miosis, anhydrosis
    B Proptosis, miosis, hyperhidrosis
    C Ptosis, mydriasis, anhydrosis
    D Ptosis, enophthalmos, hyperhidrosis
    E Proptosis, miosis, anhydrosis

10. Which virus is implicated in around 50% of cases of Hodgkin's lymphoma?

    A Human cytomegalovirus
    B Herpes simplex virus 2
    C Varicella zoster
    D Epstein–Barr virus
    E Human herpesvirus 7

11. A 54-year-old man is complaining of abdominal heaviness and short-ness of breath. On examination, his abdomen is distended, non-tender and exhibits shifting dullness with a fluid thrill. The junior doctor suspects ascites and requests a diagnostic paracentesis. It reveals a Serum-Ascites Albumin Gradient (SAAG) of 9 g/L. Which of the following is a potential cause of his ascites?

    A Cirrhosis
    B Congestive cardiac failure
    C Portal hypertension
    D Budd–Chiari syndrome
    E Nephrotic syndrome

12. A 56-year-old man has been waking up several times at night to empty his bladder. He says he doesn't feel completely empty after finishing and his stream seems to be quite 'stop and start'. He often has to strain to maintain the flow. Which of his symptoms is considered irritative?

    A Incomplete emptying
    B Having to start and stop

C Increased urination at night
D Straining
E Weak flow

13. An 8-year-old boy is brought to the GP by his mother. He has a very swollen and painful knee which arose yesterday without any preceding trauma. On closer inspection, he is afebrile and the joint, despite being swollen, does not appear inflamed. He also has several bruises across his torso. His mother mentions that her father suffered from haemophilia and that she is worried that her son may have the same disease. Blood tests are requested. Which of the following results would be suggestive of a diagnosis of haemophilia?

    A High APTT, Normal PT
    B Normal APTT, High PT
    C High APTT, High PT
    D Low bleeding time
    E Low vWF

14. An 82-year-old man is brought into A&E complaining of severe flank pain that started suddenly about 30 mins ago. On examination, he looks very unwell and his palms are cold and sweaty. Vital Signs: HR = 132 bpm; BP = 84/52 mm Hg. What is your top differential?

    A Myocardial infarction
    B Ruptured abdominal aortic aneurysm
    C Ureteric colic
    D Disc prolapse
    E Muscle sprain

15. A 31-year-old lady, who is 7 months pregnant, is brought to A&E having become extremely short of breath this morning. She has also experienced sharp chest pain on her right side. Examination reveals no abnormalities and an ECG shows sinus tachycardia. A pulmonary embolism is suspected. What is the most appropriate investigation to request?

    A D-Dimer

    B CTPA

    C VQ scan

    D Chest X-ray

    E Doppler ultrasound of the lower limbs

16. A 76-year-old woman is brought to A&E by her daughter. She is complaining of severe left iliac fossa pain accompanied by nausea, vomiting and fever. On inspection, she shows signs of peritonism. Vital signs: HR = 123 bpm, RR = 24 bpm, Temp = 38.7°C and BP = 87/54 mm Hg. An erect CXR is requested, which shows air under the diaphragm. A diagnosis of perforated diverticulitis localised to the sigmoid colon is made. What is the most appropriate surgical procedure?

    A Left colectomy

    B Abdominoperineal resection

    C Hartmann's procedure

    D Delorme procedure

    E Anterior resection

17. Which of the following tumour markers is associated with ovarian cancer?

    A CA 15-3

    B CA 19-9

    C CA 125

    D CEA

    E aFP

18. A 61-year-old man visits his GP complaining of a 'shooting pain' in his legs. The pain comes on when he walks his dog, and it gets particularly bad when walking downhill. On questioning, he reveals that he has been urinating about 10 times every day, which is much more than usual. On examination, there is a loss of sensation up to the T10 vertebral level, increased tone in his legs and brisk ankle jerks. The

GP also notices that the patient has a stooped posture. What is the most likely diagnosis?

A Benign prostate hypertrophy
B Motor neuron disease
C Sciatica
D Spinal cord stenosis
E Cauda equina syndrome

19. A 11-year-old girl, who has recently moved to the UK from Cambodia, is referred to the cardiology department after her GP identified a heart murmur a few weeks after diagnosing her with a throat infection. She has also experienced intermittent joint pain, mainly affecting her knees and hips. On examination, she has a mid-diastolic murmur heard loudest over the mitral area and a few small, mobile nodules are palpated along the ulnar border of her forearms. What is the most likely diagnosis?

A Infective endocarditis
B Rheumatic fever
C Septic arthritis
D Rheumatoid arthritis
E Lyme disease

20. A 12-year-old boy is brought into A&E — he is extremely drowsy, appears dehydrated and has vomited whilst in the ambulance. He is also clutching his abdomen and appears to be in considerable pain. He is a known diabetic, and DKA is suspected. The patient begins breathing in a very deep and laboured manner. What is the name given to this pattern of breathing?

A Cheyne–Stokes breathing
B Hypoventilation
C Kussmaul breathing
D Biot's respiration
E Apnoea

21. A 21-year-old man has been experiencing some scrotal discomfort over the past month, which he describes as feeling 'heavier than usual'. On examination, a firm, non-tender lump can be palpated at the base of the right testicle. The patient had an undescended testicle as a child, which was corrected with orchidopexy. A diagnosis of testicular cancer is suspected. The registrar recommends performing a CT scan to assess for spread. Which group of lymph nodes does testicular cancer spread to?

    A Inguinal
    B Femoral
    C Para-aortic
    D Iliac
    E Mesenteric

22. Which of the following matches the criteria for type-2 respiratory failure?

    A $PaO_2 < 10.5$ kPa, $PaCO_2 > 6$ kPa
    B $PaO_2 < 8$ kPa, $PaCO_2 > 6$ kPa
    C $PaO_2 < 10.5$ kPa, $PaCO_2 > 8$ kPa
    D $SaO_2 < 90\%$, $PaCO_2 < 8$ kPa
    E $SaO_2 < 90\%$, $PaO_2 < 8$ kPa

23. A 26-year-old model comes to see her GP after having noticed some blood streaked on the paper after emptying her bowels. This started 2 weeks ago. She adds that defecation is very painful. When asked about her diet, she reveals that she often eats ready meals and drinks relatively little water because her job involves regular travelling making it difficult for her to maintain a healthy diet. What is the most likely diagnosis?

    A Haemorrhoids
    B Anal fissure
    C Anal fistula
    D Colorectal cancer
    E Ulcerative colitis

24. A 71-year-old man presents with an 8-month history of worsening shortness of breath on exertion, orthopnoea and a cough productive of pink, frothy sputum. He has a past medical history of ischaemic heart disease and type 2 diabetes mellitus. Heart failure is suspected. What is the best investigation to confirm a diagnosis of heart failure?

    A ECG
    B Brain natriuretic peptide
    C Atrial natriuretic peptide
    D Echocardiogram
    E Chest X-ray

25. An inpatient on the respiratory ward is currently undergoing treatment for a pneumonia that he developed 2 days ago. A blood test is performed which shows a low white cell count, with a particularly low neutrophil count. The patient is re-examined and found to have a considerably enlarged spleen. On further questioning, he has suffered from three infections in the past 5 months and complains that his rheumatoid arthritis has been getting worse. What is the most likely diagnosis?

    A Malaria
    B Tuberculosis
    C Felty's syndrome
    D Lymphoma
    E Chronic lymphocytic leukaemia

26. Which stain is used when testing for TB?

    A Giemsa
    B Gram
    C India Ink
    D Sudan Black
    E Ziehl–Neelsen

27. A 60-year-old man, with a history of hypertension and type 1 diabetes mellitus, is brought to A&E by his daughter. She says that 3 hours ago, when they were eating dinner, he suddenly dropped his fork and started slurring his words. On examination, the right side of his face is drooping, muscle power is 1/5 in the right arm and 5/5 in the left; 3/5 in the right leg and 5/5 in the left. What is the most appropriate management option?

    A CT head to exclude bleed, then treatment dose of warfarin
    B CT head to exclude bleed, then give antiplatelets and perform a swallow assessment
    C CT head to exclude bleed, then IV thrombolysis
    D Control blood pressure and IV mannitol
    E Craniotomy and evacuation

28. A 42-year-old wildlife photographer returns from a 6-month trip to South Africa. He has noticed a small, dark mole on his right calf, which, he claims, has not always been there. Examination reveals an asymmetrical, dark lesion with irregular borders that measures 1 cm in diameter. Malignant melanoma is suspected and an excisional biopsy is taken and sent to the pathologist. Which feature of the histological analysis is the most useful prognostic indicator in this situation?

    A Number of mitoses
    B Surface area of lesion
    C Depth of lesion
    D Mass of lesion
    E Lymphocyte infiltration

29. An 85-year-old man is brought to A&E having been found on a roundabout in the middle of the night. He is very confused with an AMTS of 4/10. U&Es are requested, which reveal hyponatraemia (Na$^+$: 118 mmol/L (135–145)). Care is taken to increase the sodium concentration slowly. What is a major consequence of raising plasma sodium concentration too rapidly?

    A Stroke
    B Rhabdomyolysis
    C Central pontine myelinolysis
    D AKI
    E Cerebral oedema

30. Which of the following antibodies is most sensitive for primary sclerosing cholangitis?

    A AMA
    B ASLA
    C ALKM-1
    D pANCA
    E ANA

Answers

1. A

Systemic sclerosis, also known as scleroderma, is a rare disease character-ised by small blood vessel damage and fibrosis in the skin and organs. There are two types that are differentiated based on the pattern of skin involvement: limited (face and the limbs distal to the knees and elbows) and diffuse (entire body). Limited cutaneous systemic sclerosis was previ-ously known as 'CREST syndrome' because the main features of it are: **C**alcinosis, **R**aynaud's phenomenon, o**E**sophageal dysmotility, **S**clerodactyly and **T**elangiectasia.

2. B

A pneumothorax is a collection of air in the pleural space, which compro-mises the ability of the pleura to tether the lungs to the chest wall and results in partial or complete lung collapse. Pneumothoraces can be trau-matic or spontaneous (occurring without traumatic injury). A spontaneous pneumothorax can be described as primary (occurring in patients with normal lungs) or secondary (occurring in patients with prior lung disease e.g. COPD). Primary spontaneous pneumothorax is more common in tall, thin young people, like the patient described in this question. In some cases of pneumothorax, the area of pleura that is damaged can form a one-way valve resulting in the progressive accumulation of air in the pleural space — this is called a tension pneumothorax.

It is unlikely to be a PE as the patient has no obvious risk factors (e.g. long-haul travel, immobility). Asthma can cause sudden-onset breathlessness, especially during exercise, however, it is unlikely to cause 'stabbing' chest pain or to present so acutely for the first time in a 32-year-old patient.

3. D

This patient is showing signs of meningitis: severe headache, fever, neck stiffness and rash. There are two clinical signs which, although seen rela-tively rarely, often come up in SBAs. Brudzinski's sign is described in this SBA — passive flexion of the neck causes the patient to involuntarily flex their hip. To elicit Kernig's sign, the patient must be lying supine, with their hip flexed and their knee flexed at 90 degrees to the hip joint. If passive extension of the knee causes pain, this is considered Kernig's positive. Both Kernig's and Brudzinski's signs are caused by meningeal irritation.

Worsening of neurological symptoms when the body is overheated (e.g. after a warm shower) is known as Uhthoff's sign. Lhermitte's sign is when flexion of the neck causes a shooting pain running down the spine. It is sometimes referred to as 'Barber seat sign' because it can occur when bending your head down during a haircut. Both signs are associated with multiple sclerosis. Tinel's sign is a feature of carpel tunnel syndrome. Tapping the wrist at the point at which the median nerve runs under the flexor retinaculum causes pain and a tingling sensation in the area of the hand supplied by the median nerve.

4. C

Courvoisier's law states that a palpably enlarged and non-tender gallbladder in the presence of painless jaundice is unlikely to be caused by gallstones — therefore, it is likely to be due to cancer. Gallstones tend to cause a fibrotic gallbladder. A pancreatic tumour, on the other hand, will reach a point at which it obstructs the biliary tree leading to a palpably enlarged but non-tender gallbladder. This diagnosis is supported by the unintentional weight loss. The change in stool and urine colour occurs because cancer of the head of the pancreas obstructs the flow of bile from the liver into the duodenum, thereby reducing the production of stercobilin (responsible for the dark colour of stool) and urobilin (responsible for the yellow colour of urine). Most pancreatic cancers are ductal adenocarcinomas that metastasize early to regional lymph nodes and the liver. They have a poor prognosis because they tend to present late.

5. D

The management of AF depends on the clinical stability of the patient and the time between the onset of symptoms and presentation. Patients who are haemodynamically unstable, irrespective of the time of onset, require DC cardioversion. Stable patients presenting within 48 hrs of onset may be offered DC cardioversion or chemical cardioversion with flecainide or amiodarone. Flecainide is contraindicated in patients with a history of ischaemic heart disease. Stable patients presenting more than 48 hrs since onset should be anticoagulated, using low-molecular weight heparin followed by warfarin, for >3 weeks before elective cardioversion. Earlier cardioversion is possible if a transoesophageal echocardiogram shows that there are no clots within the atria. The long-term management of AF involves rate control and anticoagulation. Verapamil and bisoprolol are 1st line for rate control. Digoxin may be used in some cases. Anticoagulation is achieved with warfarin, aiming for an INR of 2–3. Patients presenting for the first time with AF will be risk stratified using the CHA_2DS_2-VASc score, to determine whether they need long-term anticoagulation. Patients with paroxysmal AF will also have a 'pill in the pocket' — sotalol or flecainide PRN.

6. A

Acute lymphoblastic leukaemia (ALL) is a bone marrow malignancy characterised by the proliferation of lymphoblasts. It is the most common malignancy of childhood. It leads to bone marrow failure (resulting in anaemia, thrombocytopaenia and leukopaenia), which manifests as fatigue, dyspnoea, easy bruising and opportunistic infections. ALL also causes organ infiltration leading to lymphadenopathy, hepatosplenomegaly, and, sometimes, testicular swelling. A blood film will show a high number of circulating lymphoblasts. Furthermore, a bone marrow aspirate or biopsy will reveal a hypercellular marrow with >20% of the cells being lymphoblasts.

All leukaemias can result in bone marrow suppression, however, AML, CLL and CML are all more common in adults. AML may manifest similarly to ALL, but tissue infiltration is less prominent. Chronic leukaemias are often asymptomatic or have a chronic history spanning months or years. Hodgkin's lymphoma is a tumour of the lymphoid cells. It is diagnosed histopathologically by the presence of Reed–Sternberg cells (binucleate lymphocytes). The main features of Hodgkin's lymphoma are a painless, enlarging neck/axilla/groin mass, lymphadenopathy that becomes painful after the ingestion of alcohol, pruritus and the B symptoms of lymphoma (fever, night sweats and weight loss).

7. C

The CURB-65 score is a clinical tool used to predict mortality in community-acquired pneumonia and it helps to determine the need for hospital admission. CURB-65 scores range from 0 to 5 and is based on the following criteria, each worth 1 point:

- **C**onfusion (AMTS < 8)
- **U**rea > 7 mmol/L
- **R**espiratory rate > 30/min
- **B**lood pressure: systolic < 90 mmHg or diastolic < 60 mmHg
- Age > 65 years

A score of 0 or 1 is associated with a very low mortality within 30 days and patients can be managed in the community. A score of 2 has a slightly higher mortality and patients should be admitted for observation and treatment as inpatients. A score of 3 or more indicates severe pneumonia with a relatively high mortality. These patients should be considered for ICU admission. This patient is over 65 years old (1 point), has a respiratory rate above 30 (1 point) and has an AMTS less than 8 (1 point). She should therefore be admitted as an inpatient.

8. C

Recurrent episodes of sweating, palpitations and anxiety in young people are classic features of phaeochromocytoma. Other possible differentials include carcinoid syndrome and insulinoma. The history of thyroid cancer, along with the current presentation of a phaeochromocytoma, suggests that this patient might have Multiple Endocrine Neoplasia Type 2A (MEN 2A) — associated with parathyroid adenomas, medullary thyroid cancer and phaeochromocytomas. Investigation of phaeochromocytoma is by measuring 24-hr urine vanillylmendelic acid (VMA), a by-product of adrenaline synthesis — a high level is consistent with a diagnosis of phaeochromocytoma. Urine metanephrine (another by-product of adrenaline synthesis) can also be measured.

Serum 17-hydroxyprogesterone levels are elevated in congenital adrenal hyperplasia, a condition that can cause precocious puberty. 24-hr urine 5-hydroxyindoleacetic acid (5-HIAA) is the main metabolite of serotonin, which is released in excess in carcinoid syndrome. Although carcinoid syndrome is a possible differential for this patient, the past medical history suggestive of MEN 2A makes phaeochromocytoma more likely. Furthermore, SBAs regarding carcinoid syndrome often mention facial 'flushing' as a buzzword.

9. A

Horner's syndrome is a condition resulting from the disruption of the sympathetic nerve pathways to the face. Causes include strokes, multiple sclerosis, Pancoast lung tumours, lymphadenopathy and carotid artery dissection. It results in a triad of ptosis, miosis and anhydrosis. Patients will also have a degree of enopthlamos.

10. D

Epstein–Barr virus (EBV) is a dsDNA virus transmitted via bodily fluids, most commonly saliva and genital secretions. Many people are infected in childhood and it is usually asymptomatic. The virus lies dormant in lymphocytes and can be reactivated when the patient becomes stressed or immunosuppressed. It is implicated in several diseases, including Hodgkin's lymphoma, Burkitt's lymphoma, glandular fever, gastric cancer and nasopharyngeal cancer. EBV infection can be confirmed via an antibody assay — IgG to EBV nuclear antigens will appear 6–12 weeks after infection and is lifelong.

11. E

The SAAG is a measurement used to help determine the cause of ascites. Equation: SAAG = [serum albumin] – [ascites albumin].

SAAG > 11 g/L is considered a high SAAG and it indicates that the ascitic fluid is transudative (low protein), which is most often due to portal hypertension. An increased hydrostatic pressure within the hepatic portal system, forces fluid out of the vasculature and into the peritoneal cavity, thereby concentrating the serum albumin. Causes of a high SAAG include cirrhosis, constrictive pericarditis, congestive cardiac failure, Budd–Chiari syndrome and hepatic venous obstruction.

SAAG < 11 g/L is considered a low SAAG and it indicates that the ascitic fluid is exudative (high protein). Nephrotic syndrome is an important exception — the ascitic fluid does not have a high protein content but it does cause a low SAAG because albumin is freely filtered through damaged glomeruli, resulting in a reduced serum albumin. Other causes of a low SAAG include malignancy, pancreatitis, infection and bowel obstruction.

12. C

BPH is an age-related disease characterised by a non-malignant increase in the size of the prostate due to cell hyperplasia. BPH causes a constellation of symptoms known as lower urinary tract symptoms (LUTS). LUTS can be divided into storage (aka irritative) and voiding (aka obstructive) symptoms and remembered using the mnemonic **FUN** (storage) **WISE** (voiding): **F**requency, **U**rgency, **N**octuria, **W**eak stream, **I**ntermittency, **S**training, incomplete **E**mptying.

13. A

There are two clotting pathways, intrinsic and extrinsic, which join to form the common clotting pathway. This results in the generation of fibrin, which promotes clot stability. The extrinsic pathway is triggered by damage to endothelial cells resulting in the release of tissue factor, which activates the clotting cascade. The intrinsic pathway is less prominent physiologically. Prothrombin time (PT) is an assay used to assess the function of the extrinsic pathway. A prolonged PT suggests that the patient is deficient in one or more components of the extrinsic and common pathways. Causes include warfarin (due to depletion of factors II, VII, IX and

X) and liver disease. The activated partial thromboplastic time (APTT) is a similar assay that assesses the function of the intrinsic and common pathways.

Haemophilia is an X-linked recessive disorder caused by a deficiency in factor VIII (Haemophilia A) or factor IX (Haemophilia B). These two factors are part of the intrinsic pathway, so haemophilia will cause a prolonged APTT. PT will be normal. Haemophilia typically presents in early childhood with spontaneous bleeding, haemarthrosis (bleeding into joint spaces), painful bleeding into muscles and excessive bleeding following trauma.

14. B

A patient presenting with sudden-onset flank pain and features of circulatory collapse (e.g. tachycardia and hypotension) should raise suspicion of a ruptured abdominal aortic aneurysm (AAA). On examination, a central pulsatile and expansile mass may be palpated. An aneurysm can be visualised with an ultrasound scan, however, it will not distinguish between an intact aneurysm and one that is leaking/ruptured. A contrast CT abdomen is needed to identify a leak. These patients require urgent referral to the vascular surgery department. Large bore IV access should be established and blood should be sent for cross-matching.

15. C

Pregnancy is an important risk factor for thromboembolic disease (e.g. PE) and caution must be taken when investigating and treating such patients. First and foremost, CTPA is unsuitable in pregnancy because the ionising radiation could harm the foetus. D-dimer is a fibrin degradation product that, despite having relatively low specificity for PE, has a high negative-predictive value. It is often used to rule out PE in patients at low risk. However, pregnant women have naturally elevated levels of D-dimer, thus producing false-positive results. Therefore, a ventilation-perfusion (VQ) scan is the best option. Chest X-rays rarely show any abnormalities in PE patients although Hampton's Hump (peripheral wedge of opacity), Westermark sign (regional oligaemia) and Fleischner sign (enlarged pulmonary artery) are sometimes mentioned in SBAs.

16. C

Perforated diverticulitis is a surgical emergency. The patient is peritonitic and is likely to progress to septic shock without treatment. Urgent removal of the affected part of the colon is required. Removal of the sigmoid colon has two main approaches. Primary anastomosis involves removal of the sigmoid colon and joining of the loose ends to form an anastomosis. This tends to be performed in the treatment of localised sigmoid tumours. A peritonitic patient is not a suitable candidate for primary anastomosis because the anastomosis is unlikely to heal under suboptimal inflammatory conditions. Given the peritonitic conditions described in this patient, a Hartmann's procedure is preferred. This involves removal of the sigmoid colon with the formation of a rectal stump and an end colostomy. It allows time for the inflammatory process to resolve and the operation can be reversed, forming an anastomosis, at a more suitable time.

A left colectomy involves removal of the colon from 2/3 of the way along the transverse colon, up to the start of the sigmoid colon. Indications include colon cancer localised to the descending colon. An abdominoperineal (AP) resection removes the anus, rectum and distal sigmoid colon — an end colostomy is formed. It is used for low-lying rectal tumours. An anterior resection removes the upper 2/3 of the rectum and part of the sigmoid colon. The anal sphincter remains intact and an anastomosis is formed. It is used for high-lying rectal tumours. Delorme's procedure is performed for full thickness rectal prolapse.

17. C

CA 15-3 = Breast cancer
CA 19-9 = Pancreatic cancer
CA 125 = Ovarian cancer
CEA = Colorectal cancer
aFP = Liver cancer, Testicular cancer (non-seminomas)
b-hCG = Choriocarcinoma, Germ cell tumours
S100 = Melanoma
Calcitonin = Medullary thyroid cancer

PSA = Prostate cancer

Thyroglobulin = Thyroid cancer (used post-thyroidectomy to monitor completeness of removal)

18. D

Spinal cord stenosis is a narrowing of the spinal canal, most commonly occurring in the lumbar spine. It can be caused by osteophytes (bony spurs that may develop in osteoarthritis and Paget's disease), disk herniation, ligamentum flavum hypertrophy, intrinsic cord tumours and trauma. The key parts of this history are the sciatica-like pain experienced when walking downhill and the patient's stooped posture. They are characteristic of spinal cord stenosis and occur because lumbar extension (e.g. when walking downhill) causes narrowing of the spinal canal and compression of the spinal cord. The pain is somewhat relieved by walking with a stooped posture or by sitting down as lumbar flexion slightly widens the spinal canal and reduces the pressure on the cord. Spinal cord compression can manifest as paresis, weakness, sensory loss, sphincter dysfunction and erectile problems.

BPH is incorrect as it does not cause any neurological deficits. Motor neuron disease can also be ruled out as it does not affect sensation. Although the pain described sounds much like sciatica, the rest of the clinical picture (mainly the effect of positional changes) points towards an alternative diagnosis. Cauda equina syndrome is a severe form of lumbar spinal stenosis caused by sudden compression of the nerves of the cauda equina. It presents acutely with urinary retention and lower back pain. Examination findings include lower motor neuron signs, perianal numbness and lax anal tone. An important distinction to take note of is that acute cord compression (such as cauda equina syndrome) causes lower motor neuron signs, whereas gradual cord compression (as in this patient) causes upper motor neuron signs.

19. B

Rheumatic fever is an infection that is becoming increasingly rare in the UK, however, it is relatively common in developing countries. It is typically preceded by a pharyngeal infection, usually caused by *S. pyogenes*. It is diagnosed using the revised Jones criteria, which is composed of major and minor criteria. The five major criteria can be remembered using the mnemonic **JONES**: **J**oints (arthritis), **O** — looks like a heart (carditis e.g. tachycardia, murmurs), subcutaneous **N**odules, **E**rythema marginatum (a rash with red, raised edges and a clear centre) and **S**ydenham's chorea (involuntary semi-purposeful movements). The minor criteria are fever, raised ESR/CRP, arthralgia, prolonged PR interval and previous rheumatic fever. Evidence of recent streptococcal infection *and* 2 major criteria *or* 1 major + 2 minor criteria is diagnostic of rheumatic fever. This patient has three major criteria (arthritis, carditis and subcutaneous nodules). The antibodies produced in rheumatic fever can cross-react with heart valve tissue, leading to permanent damage and valve dysfunction.

20. C

Kussmaul breathing is characterised by deep, sighing breaths. It is a compensatory response to severe metabolic acidosis (e.g. ketoacidosis) — the deep breaths help to blow off carbon dioxide and raise pH.

Cheyne–Stokes breathing is a cyclic breathing pattern in which breathing gets progressively deeper, then progressively shallower followed by a period of apnoea. Causes include brainstem damage or herniation. Hypoventilation broadly refers to a decrease in ventilation. Biot's respiration is characterised by clusters of rapid, shallow inspirations and expirations interspersed amongst periods of apnoea. It is also caused by brainstem damage. Apnoea refers to the temporary cessation of breathing.

21. C

Testicular tumours usually occur in young men. It may be asymptomatic and discovered during self-examination or it may cause some scrotal discomfort. The main risk factors for testicular cancer are maldescended or ectopic testes. Testicular tumours spread to the para-aortic lymph nodes. This may occasionally cause backache. Scrotal and penile tumours and infections will lead to enlargement of inguinal lymph nodes.

22. B

There are two main types of respiratory failure and they can be remembered as follows:

- Type 1 = one thing wrong = low oxygen (PaO_2 < 8 kPa, $PaCO_2$ = normal)
- Type 2 = two things wrong = low oxygen *and* high carbon dioxide (PaO_2 < 8 kPa *and* $PaCO_2$ > 6 kPa)

Type 1 respiratory failure tends to be caused by focal lung diseases (i.e. affecting only one part of the lung) such as pneumonia and PE. Type 2 respiratory failure tends to be caused by more diffuse lung diseases such as COPD and pulmonary fibrosis.

23. B

Rectal bleeding in young people is usually caused by haemorrhoids, anal fissures, coeliac disease and inflammatory bowel disease. The relationship between the blood and the stool/toilet paper is a valuable clue when distinguishing between these causes. An anal fissure is a painful tear in the squamous lining of the lower anal canal, which causes pain on defecation and bright red blood streaked on the toilet paper/stools but not mixed in with the stools. Anal fissures often occur in patients with a low fibre diet and poor fluid intake who may be constipated and strain at the stool.

Haemorrhoids are enlarged and engorged anal vascular cushions that can bleed. They are very common and usually present with bright red rectal bleeding that is separate to the stool and may drip into the pan after defecation. An anal fistula is an abnormal connection between the anus and the epithelial surface of a more proximal part of the GI tract (e.g. rectum) — this is a recognised complication of Crohn's disease. Blood is usually mixed with the stool in colorectal cancer rather than streaked on the paper. Ulcerative colitis usually causes painless rectal bleeding and may have associated symptoms such as erythema nodosum and uveitis.

24. D

An echocardiogram is the best investigation for definitively diagnosing heart failure, because it allows assessment of ventricular function and cardiac output. An echocardiogram may also provide evidence that helps identify the cause of heart failure (e.g. regional wall motion abnormalities resulting from previous infarctions, valve dysfunction, cardiomyopathy).

An ECG may also provide clues about the cause of heart failure (e.g. arrhythmias, pathological Q waves — a sign of previous MI). Brain-natriuretic peptide (BNP) is a hormone released by the ventricles in response to stretch. It stimulates natriuresis and vasodilation. Despite not being very specific, BNP is almost always raised in heart failure and has a high negative-predictive value, meaning that it is useful when ruling out heart failure. Atrial natriuretic peptide (ANP) is a similar hormone that is released by the atria in response to stretch. It also stimulates natriuresis and vasodilation, however, it is less useful as a biomarker for heart failure. Chest X-rays can reveal important signs supporting the diagnosis of heart failure — remembered as **ABCDE**: **A**lveolar shadowing, Kerley **B** lines, **C**ardiomegaly, **D**ilated upper lobe vessels, **E**ffusion.

25. C

Felty's syndrome is a triad of rheumatoid arthritis, splenomegaly and neutropenia. It most commonly occurs in patients with a history of rheumatoid arthritis, although it is possible for the rheumatoid arthritis to manifest after the other features. The low neutrophil count results in the patient suffering from frequent infections.

26. E

TB is a common topic in SBAs and Ziehl–Neelsen staining is used as a buzzword to indicate that the SBA is about TB.

The other stains are used for the following conditions/organisms:

- Giemsa – Malaria
- Gram – distinguish between differences in cell wall composition of different bacteria (*M. tuberculosis* does not respond predictably to Gram staining)

- India Ink – *Cryptococcus spp.*
- Sudan Black – Acute myeloid leukaemia

27. C

Given the acute-onset weakness and aphasia, it is likely that this patient has had a stroke. There are two main types of stroke: **ischaemic** (80%) — in which the brain is temporarily starved of blood due to thrombosis, emboli or hypotension — and **haemorrhagic** — where a bleed within the brain creates pressure that damages the brain tissue. Such bleeds may come from microaneurysm rupture, trauma, tumours, vasculitis or arteriovenous malformations. The single most important risk factor is hypertension, but others include smoking, hyperlipidaemia and diabetes. Management of ischaemic and haemorrhagic strokes differ, so an urgent CT head scan is required to distinguish between the two. Once a bleed has been excluded (by the absence of bleeding on a CT head scan), you need to determine the next stage of the management by considering the time since the onset of symptoms. If the onset of symptoms was less than 4.5 hours ago, the patient should be thrombolysed with alteplase and given aspirin within 24 hrs. If the onset of symptoms was more than 4.5 hrs ago, the patient should be given antiplatelet therapy and undergo a swallow assessment and GCS monitoring. Anticoagulation therapy is not used routinely for the treatment of ischaemic strokes. Blood pressure control and IV mannitol (used to reduce intracranial pressure) form part of the management of a haemorrhagic stroke. Craniotomy and evacuation may be performed to remove the haematoma.

28. C

Suspected melanomas are usually treated with excision biopsy (in which the entire lesion is removed, unlike a core biopsy in which only a section of the tissue is sampled). Histopathologists will measure the depth of penetration of the melanoma — known as the Breslow thickness. This is a very useful prognostic indicator in melanoma. The other options have no association with prognosis in melanoma.

29. C

Central pontine myelinolysis (CPM) is a neurological condition caused by damage to the myelin sheath of the neurons that make up the pons. It manifests as acute paralysis, dysarthria and dysphagia. Cells of the central nervous system adjust their intracellular ion concentrations in response to serum osmolality. In patients with chronic hyponatraemia, their myelin cells will compensate by decreasing their intracellular ion concentration, so that they remain isotonic in their environment — thereby preventing the absorption of excess fluid. When hyponatraemia is corrected gradually, the extracellular osmolality increases slowly and the intracellular ion concentration within the myelin cells will be able to increase in accordance with this change. When the correction is too rapid, the brain cells do not have enough time to adapt to the increasing extracellular osmolality and the osmotic gradient between the myelin cells and the extracellular environment will draw water out of the myelin cells, ultimately resulting in CPM.

30. D

Primary sclerosing cholangitis (PSC) is T-cell mediated autoimmune destruction of the extrahepatic and intrahepatic biliary ducts, leading to multifocal scarring. It can progress to cirrhosis and end-stage liver failure. Although often asymptomatic and diagnosed based on incidental findings, symptoms may include jaundice, pruritus, weight loss, right upper quadrant pain, dark urine, pale faeces and a history of ulcerative colitis (there is a strong association between PSC and UC). Liver function tests would show elevated ALP, AST and ALT and serology is likely to be positive for perinuclear anti-neutrophil cytoplasmic antibodies (pANCA). An abdominal ultrasound will show abnormal bile ducts and ERCP/MRCP will show multi-focal intrahepatic and extra-hepatic strictures and dilations.

pANCA is very sensitive for PSC — 80% of PSC patients test positive. It can, however, be elevated in other conditions, such as microscopic polyangiitis, granulomatosis with polyangiitis and rheumatoid arthritis. ANA is also positive in up to 50% of patients with PSC, but is less specific. AMA is detected in 95% of patients with primary biliary cirrhosis (PBC). ASLA and ALKM-1 are seen in type 1 and type 2 autoimmune hepatitis, respectively.

Paper 6

Questions

1. Which of the following is not a sign of cirrhosis?

    A Gynaecomastia
    B Asterixis
    C Koilonychia
    D Hepatic fetor
    E Clubbing

2. A 67-year-old pensioner, with a 40 pack-year smoking history, visits his GP complaining of shortness of breath that has gradually been getting worse over the past 6 months. He used to be able to walk 500 m to the shops but now he struggles to make it up the stairs at home. He has also been suffering from a persistent cough productive of clear sputum. Which investigation is required to confirm the diagnosis?

    A Spirometry
    B Peak expiratory flow
    C Sputum culture
    D Chest X-ray
    E Bronchoscopy and biopsy

3. An 18-year-old man visits the GP having recently returned from a holiday to Thailand. He complains of a 2-day history of watery, bloody diarrhoea and has vomited six times. On examination, he is pyrexial with diffuse abdominal tenderness. Which organism is most likely to be causing his symptoms?

    A *Giardia lamblia*
    B *Vibrio cholera*
    C Norovirus
    D *E. coli* O157
    E *Salmonella*

4. A 42-year-old man is brought into A&E by his wife. He is clutching his head and appears to be drowsy and distressed. Though a clear history is difficult to ascertain, he mentions that he has an 'absolutely devastating headache' that suddenly came on this morning. He has never experienced pain like this before. Towards the end of the consultation, he begins to vomit. He is apyrexial and denies any trauma to the head. On examination, the patient's neck is slightly stiff, he is hypertensive and has large bilateral palpable masses in his abdomen. On direct questioning, he reveals that his father died suddenly at the age of 49. Which underlying disease has predisposed the patient to this clinical scenario?

    A Renal cell carcinoma
    B Polycystic kidney disease
    C Medullary sponge kidney
    D Phaeochromocytoma
    E Subdural haemorrhage

5. A 33-year-old man has recently been diagnosed with hypertension following the incidental finding of abnormally high blood pressure during a routine check-up at his GP practice. Without further investigation, he was started on Ramipril. 1 week later, he begins to feel very nauseous and vomits several times. He is taken to A&E where his renal function is monitored:

    Urea: 8.1 mmol/L (2.5–6.7)
    Creatinine: 240 — mmol/L (baseline: 102)
    eGFR: 53 ml/min/1.73 m^2 (> 90)
    Urine output: 20 mL/hr (> 0.5 mL/kg/hr)

What is the most likely cause of his condition?

    A Acute tubular necrosis
    B Acute interstitial nephritis
    C Glomerulonephritis
    D Renal artery stenosis
    E Vasculitis

6. A 47-year-old man comes to A&E having experienced palpitations. He has a past medical history of hypertension which is being treated with ramipril and spironolactone. An ECG shows tented T waves and flattened P waves. A blood test reveals:

    Na^+: 137 mmol/L (135–145)
    K^+: 6.8 mmol/L (3.5–5)
    Ca^{2+}: 2.3 mmol/L (2.2–2.6)
    pH: 7.35 (7.35–7.45)

What is the first step in the management of this patient?

    A IV salbutamol
    B 50 ml 50% dextrose with 10U insulin
    C 50 ml 5% dextrose with 10U insulin
    D 10 ml 10% calcium gluconate
    E IV sodium bicarbonate

7. Whilst eating dinner with his family, an 11-year-old boy suddenly drops his cutlery and begins to stare blankly into space. His eyelids begin to flutter, his eyes roll upwards and this continues for 10 s. His dad notices the event and asks him about it, but he can't remember what happened. What type of seizure is this describing?

    A Absence
    B Simple partial
    C Complex partial
    D Myoclonic
    E Atonic

8. A 71-year-old man has had a 2-week history of shortness of breath that improves when lying flat. On examination, the patient has an oxygen saturation of 88%, his fingers are clubbed and there are multiple spider naevi on his chest. Shifting dullness is demonstrated, his spleen is enlarged and there are dilated veins around his umbilicus. The patient has a history of alcohol abuse. What is the most likely diagnosis?

   A Congestive cardiac failure
   B Portal hypertension
   C Hepatopulmonary syndrome
   D GI bleed
   E Alcoholic hepatitis

9. A 72-year-old man is admitted to the orthopaedic surgery ward after fracturing his distal humerus whilst gardening. He mentioned that he suddenly felt a severe pain in his right arm and denies any significant preceding trauma. He adds that he has recently been urinating a lot more frequently (often up to 12 times per day) and has suffered from constipation, which he attributes to being 'part of growing old'. An X-ray of the affected arm reveals a pathological fracture with lytic deposits throughout the bone.

   Blood tests reveal:
   ESR = 48 mm/hr (0–22)
   Ca^{2+} = 3.1 mmol/L (2.2–2.6)

   What is the most likely diagnosis?

   A Multiple myeloma
   B Paget's disease
   C Osteoporosis
   D Vitamin D deficiency
   E Thyrotoxicosis

10. A 49-year-old man is referred to the respiratory department by his GP. He has been suffering from gradual-onset, worsening shortness of breath over the past 3 months. His 50 pack-year smoking history

makes COPD the top differential. Spirometry confirms these suspicions. What is the most appropriate first step in the pharmacological management of this patient?

A Inhaled corticosteroid
B Inhaled ipratropium bromide
C Inhaled tiotropium
D Symbicort
E Long-term oxygen therapy

11. Which of the following is a sign of a lower motor neuron lesion?

A Hyperreflexia
B Spasticity
C Fasciculations
D Clonus
E Babinski's sign

12. A 47-year-old man has been suffering from rhinitis and recurrent nosebleeds for the past 3 months. At first, he attributed this to the cold weather, however, over the last 3 weeks he has started coughing up a small amount of blood. A series of bedside tests are performed, including a urine dipstick, which reveals proteinuria and haematuria. Blood tests and antibody screens reveal a raised ESR and cANCA. What is the most likely diagnosis?

A Microscopic polyangiitis
B Goodpasture's syndrome
C Granulomatosis with polyangiitis
D Churg–Strauss syndrome
E Behçet's disease

13. Which of the following organisms most commonly causes gas gangrene?

A *Streptococcus pyogenes*
B *Staphylococcus aureus*

    C *Staphylococcus epidermidis*
    D *Clostridium perfringens*
    E *Haemophilus influenzae*

14. A 16-year-old schoolgirl books an appointment with her GP after noticing a lump in her left breast during self-examination. She, sensibly, decided to seek medical attention. She complains of no other symptoms. On examination, a 1 cm × 1 cm firm, smooth and very mobile lump is palpated in the upper-outer quadrant of her left breast. There is no pain on palpation nor is there any axillary or cervical lymphadenopathy. What is the most likely diagnosis?

    A Fibrocystic disease
    B Fibroadenoma
    C Breast cancer
    D Breast abscess
    E Fat necrosis

15. Which of the following drug classes is most likely to cause iatrogenic hypoglycaemia in diabetes patients?

    A Sulfonylureas
    B Metformin
    C Glucagon
    D Hydrocortisone
    E Orlistat

16. A 24-year-old swimwear model presents to A&E with severe right iliac fossa pain. The pain was initially poorly localised to the umbilical region, before moving to the right iliac fossa. This has been accompanied by nausea, anorexia and fever. A diagnosis of appendicitis is made and she is referred for an appendicectomy. What is the most suitable surgical incision for this patient?

    A Lanz
    B Kocher

C Pfannenstiel
D Rutherford-Morrison
E Gridiron

17. A 55-year-old man presents to his GP having coughed up blood on several occasions over the past 6 months. He said that he has had a 'smokers' cough' for years but the appearance of blood has been a recent change. On direct questioning, he admits to unintentionally losing about 5 kg of weight over the past 6 months. A chest X-ray shows a 2 cm cavitating lesion in the right upper lobe. There appears to be a few other smaller nodules surrounding the large cavitating lesion. The left lung appears slightly fibrosed, but is otherwise normal. What is the most likely diagnosis?

   A Small cell lung cancer
   B Squamous cell lung cancer
   C Atypical pneumonia
   D Lung abscess
   E Goodpasture's syndrome

18. A 46-year-old airline pilot presents to A&E with severe pain in his right flank. He adds that the pain moves down towards his right groin. Though examination is difficult, as he is writhing around in pain, no abnormalities are detected. However, a urine dipstick reveals haematuria. Which investigation would you do next?

   A Renal ultrasound
   B Cystoscopy
   C CT-KUB
   D MRI
   E Urine MC&S

19. A 32-year-old man, with a history of IV drug abuse, presents to A&E with a high fever and rigors. He has also been very breathless and has experienced epigastric pain that is worse on exertion. On

examination, giant V waves are seen in the JVP and tender, pulsatile hepatomegaly is palpated. What is the most likely diagnosis?

    A Mitral stenosis
    B Tricuspid regurgitation
    C Pulmonary hypertension
    D Portal hypertension
    E Viral hepatitis

20. A 31-year-old female presents to her GP with a 2-month history of fatigue and worsening muscle weakness. She also complains that her left eyelid droops considerably more than her right. She feels fine in the morning but her strength decreases throughout the day, especially if she exerts herself more so than usual. Myasthenia gravis is suspected. Which of the following investigations may provide evidence supporting this diagnosis?

    A Dix–Hallpike test
    B Schirmer's test
    C Romberg's test
    D Tensilon test
    E Trendelenberg test

21. A 15-year-old school boy is rushed into A&E having accidentally ingested some peanuts, to which he is extremely allergic. His face and lips are swollen, he is wheezing and struggling to breathe. Vital signs: HR = 132 bpm, BP = 88/53 mm Hg. His airway has been secured and he is being given 100% oxygen. What is the next most appropriate step in the management of this patient?

    A IV chlorpheniramine
    B IV hydrocortisone
    C IV saline
    D IV adrenaline
    E IM adrenaline

22. Which of the following is a cause of microcytic anaemia?

    A Myelodysplasia
    B Multiple myeloma
    C Thalassaemia
    D Myelofibrosis
    E Aplastic anaemia

23. A 63-year-old type 2 diabetic presents with a rash on her shins that has gradually got worse over the past 3 months. On closer inspection, there are three areas of raised, reddened and hardened skin with a yellowish centre. What is the most likely diagnosis?

    A Acanthosis nigricans
    B Diabetic dermopathy
    C Necrobiosis lipoidica diabeticorum
    D Granuloma annulare
    E Pruritus

24. A 76-year-old woman is brought into A&E with central crushing chest pain that radiates to her jaw and left arm. An ECG is performed, which shows ST elevation in leads ll, lll and aVF. Her SaO_2 is 90%. Before she is sent to the cathlab for percutaneous coronary intervention, she is started on a combination of drugs. Which of the following should not be given?

    A Morphine
    B Oxygen
    C Aspirin
    D Clopidogrel
    E Warfarin

25. A 42-year-old amateur rugby player presents to his GP complaining that his teammates have been making fun of his 'man boobs'. He admits that he appears to have developed breasts over the past few months and it is causing him considerable embarrassment and

distress. Which of the following drugs is most likely to have caused this unfortunate circumstance?

A Cimetidine
B Aspirin
C Salbutamol
D Ramipril
E Omeprazole

26. Which part of the prostate gland undergoes progressive hyperplasia in BPH?

A Central zone
B Transitional zone
C Peripheral zone
D Ejaculatory duct
E Anterior fibromuscular stroma

27. A 62-year-old obese man visits his GP complaining of a cramping pain in his buttocks that comes on when he walks his Pomeranian, Skippy. This pain was first noticed 4 months ago and it is relieved by sitting down. He has a 40 pack-year smoking history. On direct questioning, he sheepishly admits to suffering from erectile dysfunction over the last 2 months. Examination is normal except for noticeably weak pedal pulses. What is the most likely diagnosis?

A Chronic compartment syndrome
B Leriche syndrome
C Critical limb ischaemia
D Spinal stenosis
E Chronic deep vein thrombosis

28. A 43-year-old man, who has recently moved to the UK from Greece, has been referred for an outpatient appointment to discuss his recurrent mouth ulcers. He says that, for the past 8 months, he has regularly

suffered from oral ulcers and he, quite timidly, mentions that he has also noticed ulcers on his penis. During the consultation, you notice that his eyes look quite red. When asked about it, he mentions that his eyes have been very itchy and painful recently, but attributes this to hay fever. What is the most likely diagnosis?

A Inflammatory bowel disease
B Behçet's disease
C Herpes simplex virus
D Syphilis
E Reactive arthritis

29. Which of the following ECG findings is associated with pulmonary embolism?

A Bradycardia
B Tall tented T waves
C Reverse tick sign
D S1Q3T3
E T wave inversion

30. Which of the following is not a feature of Parkinson's disease?

A Hypomimia
B Hypophonia
C Micrographia
D Furrowed eyebrows
E Wide-based gait

Answers

1. C

There are several signs associated with liver failure. They can be remembered as the A to J of liver failure: **A**sterixis, **B**ruising, **C**lubbing, **D**upuytren's contracture, **E**rythema (palmar), **F**etor hepaticus, **G**ynaecomastia, **H**epatomegaly (in early cirrhosis), **I**tching and **J**aundice. Other examination findings include spider naevi, leukonychia, testicular atrophy and signs of portal hypertension, such as splenomegaly, GI bleeds, caput medusae, haemorrhoids and ascites. Koilonychia is spooning of the nails which occurs due to chronic iron deficiency. It is associated with Plummer–Vinson syndrome — a disease characterised by the formation of oesophageal webs leading to dysphagia.

2. A

This SBA describes a typical COPD patient — extensive smoking history, worsening shortness of breath and a cough productive of clear sputum. N.B. During an infective exacerbation of COPD, the sputum may become green/yellow. COPD is diagnosed using spirometry to measure FEV1 and FVC. An FEV1 <80% predicted (sometimes shown as <0.8) and an FEV1/FVC ratio <0.7, which does not improve or improves very little with the administration of bronchodilators, is diagnostic of COPD. A chest X-ray may be performed which might show hyperinflated lungs (>6 anterior ribs seen above the diaphragm), however, spirometry is the gold standard investigation.

Peak expiratory flow is used to monitor asthma. A sputum culture will be useful in patients showing signs of respiratory infection. Bronchoscopy and biopsy is used to diagnose lung cancer, interstitial lung disease and infiltrative diseases of the lungs (e.g. sarcoidosis).

3. D

A short history of diarrhoea and vomiting with a fever and abdominal tenderness is suggestive of gastroenteritis. There are five common organisms which cause bloody diarrhoea — the '**CHESS**' organisms: *C*ampylobacter jejuni, **H**aemorrhagic *E. coli* (O157), *E*ntamoeba histol-ytica, **S**almonella and **S**higella. *E. coli* (O157) is the most common cause of travellers' diarrhoea and, given that this patient has recently returned from his travels to Thailand, it is the most likely causative organism.

Salmonella is usually acquired by ingestion of contaminated poultry. Norovirus is the winter vomiting bug. It is very contagious, often spread-ing through schools. It causes diarrhoea, however, nausea and vomiting are the predominant features. Vibrio cholerae is spread via the faecal-oral route and classically produces 'rice-water stools'. Giardia is a parasite that causes giardiasis. It presents with non-bloody diarrhoea, abdominal cramps and foul-smelling flatulence and belching.

4. B

A sudden onset 'worst headache ever' is the classic presentation of suba-rachnoid haemorrhage. It may be accompanied by nausea, vomiting, neck stiffness and reduced consciousness. It is an emergency and requires urgent neurosurgical assessment. Polycystic kidney disease is an autosomal domi-nant condition that results in bilaterally enlarged kidneys, hypertension and haematuria. It is strongly associated with subarachnoid haemorrhage (though the mechanism is unclear). Some patients with polycystic kidney disease may have a family history of sudden death (from subarachnoid haemorrhages). Other conditions predisposing to subarachnoid haemor-rhage include Marfan's syndrome and Ehlers–Danlos syndrome.

Subdural haemorrhage tends to occur following head trauma. A gradually enlarging collection of blood between the dura and arachnoid mater leads to fluctuating consciousness and worsening neurological symptoms (e.g. headache, focal weakness and confusion). Subdural haemorrhages can be considered acute, subacute or chronic based on the interval between pres-entation and head trauma. Renal cell carcinoma usually presents with a triad of loin pain, palpable abdominal mass (although this is unlikely to be bilateral) and haematuria.

5. D

When young people get diagnosed with hypertension, secondary causes should always be considered and investigated appropriately. Renal artery stenosis is a cause of secondary hypertension. The reduced blood flow to the kidneys in renal artery stenosis is compensated by angiotensin II-mediated constriction of the efferent arteriole, which maintains pressure across the glomerulus. ACE inhibitors reduce the production of angiotensin II, thereby reducing its vasoconstrictive effect on the efferent arteriole resulting in a drop in the pressure across the glomerulus and, hence, glomerular filtration rate. This leads to AKI (as seen in this patient). For this reason, ACE inhibitors are contraindicated in bilateral renal artery stenosis.

Acute tubular necrosis (ATN) is one of the most common causes of AKI and usually results from pre-renal (e.g. hypovolaemia) or intrinsic renal (e.g. nephrotoxic drugs) issues. As tubular cells continually replace themselves, patients often recover from ATN within a few days/weeks. Acute interstitial nephritis (AIN) is a type of nephritis that is usually caused by an adverse reaction to a drug. Symptoms of AIN include a fever, rash, nausea and vomiting.

6. D

Hyperkalaemia is a serious electrolyte abnormality. As potassium is important in the generation of the cardiac action potential, hyperkalameia can lead to life-threatening arrhythmias. Signs and symptoms of hyperkalaemia include general muscle weakness, flaccid paralysis, paraesthesia of the hands and feet, lethargy, confusion and palpitations. This patient's hyperkalaemia is likely to be an adverse effect of spironolactone (potassium-sparing diuretic). Hyperkalaemia causes several distinctive ECG changes. They tend to occur at different degrees of hyperkalaemia:

- Tented T waves — $K^+ > 5.5$ mmol/L
- Flattening of P waves — $K^+ > 6.5$ mmol/L
- Widening of the QRS complex and bradycardia — $K^+ > 7.5$ mmol/L

Management of hyperkalaemia is performed in two steps:

1. **10 ml 10% calcium gluconate** — stabilises the myocardium and protects against arrhythmias but does not lower serum potassium levels
2. **50 ml of 50% dextrose with 10 U insulin** — insulin drives potassium into cells and dextrose is also given to prevent hypoglycaemia

Other agents that are sometimes used to treat hyperkalaemia include salbutamol nebulisers, IV sodium bicarbonate and calcium resonium.

7. A

This patient has just suffered from an absence seizure, a form of generalised seizure. Generalised seizures occur in both hemispheres of the brain and come in multiple forms. Absence seizures, often known as petit mal, begin abruptly and without warning. The patient may look as though they are daydreaming or they may make repetitive movements such as rhythmic blinking or chewing. Absence seizures also end abruptly, usually after just a few seconds and the patient will have no recollection of the episode. Another form of generalised seizure is the tonic-clonic seizure. This seizure presents itself in two stages, the initial stage is the 'tonic' phase where the person will lose consciousness and go stiff, often falling to the floor. The second, 'clonic' phase can present with jerking limbs, loss of bladder control or difficulty breathing. The patient may also bite the inside of their mouth as a result of the clonic stage. Tonic-clonic seizures should only last a few minutes, the patient will often proceed to feel exhausted and confused. Tonic and clonic seizures can also occur individually. Tonic seizures will involve stiffness but no muscle jerking and clonic seizures will present with the opposite. Another form of generalised seizure is the myoclonic seizure which often occurs just after a person has woken up. This causes the patient to exhibit muscle jerking but only for a fraction of a second. Although myoclonic seizures occur momentarily a person will often experience many of them in a short space of time, this is known as a cluster. Lastly there are atonic seizures which are the opposite of tonic seizures. Instead of stiffening, the patient will relax and appear 'floppy', often collapsing to the floor.

8. C

This patient presented with signs of portal hypertension (ascites, spleno-megaly and caput medusae). However, this is not the best answer as his presenting complaint is shortness of breath, which cannot be explained by portal hypertension alone. His portal hypertension is likely to be due to liver cirrhosis given the signs mentioned (spider naevi and clubbing) and alcohol history. A rare complication of cirrhosis is hepatopulmonary syn-drome (HPS), characterised by hypoxaemia in patients with portal hyper-tension. HPS results from microscopic pulmonary vasodilation due to decreased hepatic clearance of vasodilators. This vasodilation leads to hyperperfusion of the lungs and hypoxaemia. Because this tends to occur at the lung bases, it is common for patients to report platypnoea (dyspnoea relieved by lying flat). Congestive cardiac failure, on the other hand, causes orthopnoea (dyspnoea that is worse when lying flat).

A chronic GI bleed secondary to portal hypertension (e.g. oesophageal or rectal variceal) could cause dyspnoea due to anaemia, but it would not be affected by body position. Despite the history of alcohol abuse, alcoholic hepatitis is unlikely as it would not cause dyspnoea.

9. A

Multiple myeloma is a haematological malignancy characterised by the proliferation of plasma cells. It is associated with lytic bone lesions and excess production of a monoclonal immunoglobulin. Presenting symp-toms include bone pain, pathological fractures, recurrent infections and features of hypercalcaemia (e.g. polyuria, polydipsia and constipation). Biochemically, multiple myeloma will feature a raised ESR and serum Ca^{2+}. Serum electrophoresis will reveal a thin, dense band representing the proliferation of a monoclonal immunoglobulin. Bence-Jones proteins, which are monoclonal immunoglobulin light chains, can be detected in the urine of patients with multiple myeloma.

Osteoporosis can result in pathological fractures, but it does not affect serum biochemistry. Paget's disease causes lytic bone lesions and pathological fractures, however, it also does not affect serum biochemistry.

10. B

Like asthma, the pharmacological management of COPD has a set of guidelines constructed by the British Thoracic Society (BTS). These guidelines have been simplified below:

1. Short-acting muscarinic antagonist (SAMA e.g. ipratropium) or short-acting beta-agonist (SABA e.g. salbutamol) PRN
2. Add long-acting muscarinic antagonist (LAMA e.g. tiotropium) or long-acting beta-agonist (LABA e.g. salmeterol)
3. Consider using a LAMA + LABA or LABA with an inhaled corticosteroid (ICS)
   - Symbicort = Budesonide (ICS) + Formoterol (LABA)
4. Consider LAMA + LABA + ICS
   - General Advice to Patients: stop smoking, encourage exercise, address poor nutrition, offer influenza and pneumococcal vaccinations and pulmonary rehabilitation.

11. C

Upper and lower motor neuron lesions have very distinct, and sometimes opposite, features so it is important to be able to distinguish them confidently. Upper motor neuron (UMN) lesions (e.g. a stroke) will have an acute phase during which you get 'loss of function' signs (e.g. flaccid paralysis). Then, there will be an increase in abnormal motor function caused by the loss of descending inhibitory inputs from the central nervous system. This results in increased muscle tone (spasticity), hyperreflexia, clonus and Babinski's sign. There will be no muscle atrophy because the lower motor neurons (LMN), which are still intact, are responsible for supplying the muscles with nutrients. However, over time there will be a degree of muscle atrophy due to disuse.

LMN lesions have the opposite features: hypotonia, hyporeflexia and muscle atrophy. They also cause fasciculations and fibrillations. Fasciculations are visible twitches in the muscle, caused by damaged motor units firing spontaneous, uncoordinated action potentials. Fibrillations are twitches of individual muscle fibres that can be observed using electromyography but are not visible to the naked eye. Features of UMN and LMN lesions can co-exist in amyotrophic lateral sclerosis (ALS).

12. C

Granulomatosis with polyangiitis (GPA), previously known as Wegener's granulomatosis, is a small- and medium-vessel vasculitis which follows a classic triad of organ involvement: upper respiratory tract (nosebleeds), lungs (haemoptysis) & kidneys (glomerulonephritis). Other features include rhinitis, the 'saddle-nose' deformity and purpura. cANCA is elevated in about 90% of patients but is not specific to GPA. As it is a chronic, systemic inflammatory disease, ESR is usually raised.

Microscopic polyangiitis is a similar disease, with skin, lung and kidney involvement, but without evidence of granulomatous disease. Goodpasture's syndrome is characterised by the presence anti-GBM (glomerular basement membrane) antibodies and primarily affects the lungs and kidneys. Churg–Strauss syndrome (aka eosinophilic granulomatosis with polyangiitis) is a triphasic vasculitis consisting of an allergic phase (asthma/allergic rhinitis), eosinophilic phase (high eosinophils) and vasculitic phase (organ involvement e.g. myocardial inflammation and reduced blood flow to the heart can result in death). Behçet's disease is a small-vessel vasculitis characterised by a triad of oral ulcers, genital ulcers and uveitis.

13. D

Gangrene is tissue death due to poor vascular supply and is a feature of critical limb ischaemia. Subtypes of gangrene include wet gangrene (infection of the necrotic tissue), dry gangrene (necrosis without infection), and gas gangrene (infection that produces gas within gangrenous tissues, most commonly caused by *C. perfringens*). Gas gangrene causes large, black sores that often have necrotic bullae (large blisters). Crepitus may be heard due to escaping gas. *C. perfringens* is found in soil and enters through wounds, producing an exotoxin which destroys surrounding tissues and generates gas.

S. pyogenes and *S. aureus* are causes of necrotising fasciitis, a subtype of gangrene which destroys soft tissues. *S. pyogenes* and *S. aureus* are also responsible for most cases of cellulitis with *H. influenzae* being a common cause of orbital cellulitis. *S. epidermidis* is a normal skin commensal, however, it can cause hospital-acquired infections by forming biofilms on catheters and surgical implants.

14. B

A fibroadenoma is a benign breast tumour involving epithelial and stromal tissue. They are very common, especially in young women. On palpation, they will often feel firm, well demarcated and very mobile (hence why it is sometimes referred to as a 'breast mouse'). In a young patient with a lump matching the above description, no cervical lymphadenopathy or systemic signs of malignancy, a diagnosis of fibroadenoma is very likely. An ultrasound scan and a fine needle aspiration/biopsy should be requested to confirm the diagnosis.

15. A

Sulfonylureas are used in the treatment of type 2 diabetes mellitus (T2DM). They act by stimulating the release of insulin from beta cells in the pancreas. As they work by increasing insulin release, they can cause hypoglycaemia if the amount of insulin released is greater than the amount required to maintain a normal blood glucose.

Metformin is a biguanide that is widely used in T2DM. It increases cellular sensitivity to insulin, but does not increase insulin secretion itself — therefore, it does not cause hypoglycaemia. Glucagon and hydro-cortisone increase blood glucose levels. Orlistat inhibits pancreatic lipases and is sometimes used as an anti-obesity medication.

16. A

Lanz and Gridiron (also known as McBurney's incision) incisions can both be used when performing an appendicectomy. The Lanz incision runs along the bikini line and is preferred in patients who are particularly concerned about the cosmetic appearance of the scar (e.g. a swimwear model). It runs along body contours and is less visible than the Gridiron incision, however, they are associated with an increased risk of inguinal hernias as the incision severs the ilioinguinal and iliohypogastric nerves which innervate the muscles of the posterior wall of the inguinal canal. Gridiron incisions occur at McBurney's point and run perpendicular to a line between the ASIS and the umbilicus.

The following incisions are typically used for these operations listed below. Please bear in mind that surgical approaches are not always consistent, so do not attempt to guess an operation based on the scar.

> Right Kocher — Open Cholecystectomy
> Left Kocher — Splenectomy
> Pfannenstiel — Caesarian Section, Gynaecological Operations
> Rutherford-Morrison (also known as hockey stick incision) — Renal Transplant.

17. B

Haemoptysis and unintentional weight loss in a heavy smoker should raise suspicion of lung cancer. Squamous cell carcinoma is a type of non-small cell lung cancer, which is associated with cavitating lesions.

Small cell lung cancer is more common in smokers, however, it is not associated with cavitating lesions. Atypical pneumonia typically causes a dry cough with vague symptoms of malaise and lethargy. Lung abscesses form when the immune system fails to clear an infection. It often causes a cough productive of purulent mucus, swinging fevers and night sweats. Goodpasture's syndrome is an autoimmune condition that results in acute glomerulonephritis and lung damage (which can manifest as haemoptysis).

18. C

Excruciating 'loin to groin' pain is the textbook presentation of ureteric colic. This occurs when a stone gets stuck either in the renal pelvis or the ureter leading to strong peristaltic contractions of the ureter in an attempt to relieve the obstruction. The management of this condition depends on the size of the stone. Stones <5 mm in diameter will be left to pass spontaneously. Patients are encouraged to retain the stone, if possible, so that it can be sent for analysis which could help identify an underlying cause (e.g. hyperuricaemia leading to uric acid stones). Stones >5 mm will require surgical intervention. Procedures such as percutaneous nephrolithotomy (PCNL), extracorporeal shock wave lithotripsy (ESWL) and ureteroscopic lithotripsy can be used to relieve an obstruction. The best investigation for ureteric colic is a non-contrast CT-KUB (kidneys, ureters and bladder).

Renal ultrasound may be performed in a patient who is at high risk of forming ureteric stones (e.g. hyperparathyroidism) to check for the presence of asymptomatic stones. Cystoscopy tends to be performed to look for lesions in the bladder such as bladder tumours. MRI is unlikely to be particularly helpful in this scenario and it will be more expensive and time-consuming than a CT-KUB. Urine MC&S is performed in patients with suspected UTI to identify the causative organism.

19. B

In the presence of an incompetent tricuspid valve, ventricular contraction pushes a column of blood through the valve and right atrium up the superior vena cava, appearing as 'giant V waves' in the JVP. The backflow of blood from the right side of the heart down the inferior vena cava, due to tricuspid regurgitation, leads to hepatic venous congestion and tender, pulsatile hepatomegaly. Other features of tricuspid regurgitation include pansystolic murmur heard loudest at the lower left sternal edge during inspiration, parasternal heave, ascites and ankle oedema. The fever alongside the recent-onset cardiac symptoms in a known IV drug user makes infective endocarditis (most common cause of tricuspid regurgitation) very likely.

20. D

The Tensilon test involves administering edrophonium bromide, a very short-acting anticholinergic, and observing the patient's response. A dramatic, yet short-lived, improvement in the patient's clinical features is suggestive of myasthenia gravis. However, the Tensilon test is rarely used because it runs the risk of causing bradycardia.

The Dix–Hallpike test is used to identify benign paroxysmal positional vertigo (BPPV). Schirmer's test assesses tear production and is used to diagnose Sjögren's syndrome. Romberg's test assesses a patient's ability to maintain balance whilst standing still, thereby assessing proprioception and vestibular function. During a Trendelenburg test, a patient is asked to stand on each leg in turn to identify weak or paralysed hip abductor muscles.

21. E

This is a case of anaphylaxis — an acute condition characterised by the sudden release of vasoactive cytokines (mainly histamine) from mast cells. It often presents with shortness of breath, wheezing, swelling of the lips/face and a rash. In the immediate management of a patient in anaphylaxis, an ABC approach should be adopted. The patient's airway should be secured, and 100% oxygen should be delivered. Intubation may be considered in the case of significant airway obstruction. IM adrenaline is administered as the first step in the pharmacological management of anaphylaxis. IV adrenaline is used in cardiac arrest but not anaphylaxis. Once IV access is secured, IV chlorpheniramine (antihistamine) and IV hydrocortisone (steroid) is given. IV saline may be needed depending on the patient's blood pressure. Pulse oximetry, ECG and blood pressure should be monitored whilst the patient is recovering.

22. C

A useful mnemonic for remembering the causes of microcytic anaemia is **TAILS**: **T**halassaemia, **A**naemia of chronic disease, **I**ron deficiency, **L**ead poisoning and **S**ideroblastic anaemia (an abnormality of haem synthesis resulting in the inability to incorporate iron into haemoglobin).

Myelodysplasia and multiple myeloma are both causes of macrocytic anaemia. Other causes include vitamin B12 and folate deficiencies, alcohol excess, hypothyroidism, liver disease and haemolysis. Myelofibrosis and aplastic anaemia cause normocytic anaemia. A mnemonic for remembering the causes of normocytic anaemia is **MR I CALM**: **M**arrow failure, **R**enal failure, **I**ron deficiency (early), anaemia of **C**hronic disease (early), **A**plastic anaemia (and acute blood loss), **L**eukaemia and **M**yelofibrosis.

23. C

All the options are associated with diabetes mellitus, however, the description most closely matches necrobiosis lipoidica diabeticorum. Acanthosis nigricans is an area of dark, velvety skin usually found in body folds (e.g. axilla). It is associated with several endocrine conditions, such as type 2 diabetes mellitus, Cushing's syndrome and polycystic ovarian syndrome. It can also occur as a paraneoplastic syndrome due to gastrointestinal cancers. Diabetic dermopathy is characterised by slightly depressed reddish-brown patches that most frequently occur on the shins. Granuloma annulare is a peculiar skin condition that looks like a ring of pink-purple skin lumps most often found on the backs of the hands and feet. It is associated with diabetes mellitus and thyroid disease; however, it can occur spontaneously in normal people. 'Pruritus' is a non-specific medical term for 'itching'.

24. E

Acutely, all patients with acute coronary syndrome are started on a combination of medications, which can be remembered with the mnemonic **MONABASH**:

- **M**orphine sulphate/diamorphine (often given with an anti-emetic like metoclopramide to help deal with the nausea caused by morphine)
- **O**xygen: aiming for a saturation >94%
- **N**itrates: GTN or isosorbide mononitrate
- **A**ntiplatelets: aspirin and clopidogrel
- **B**eta-blockers: to reduce myocardial oxygen demand.

Contraindicated in patients with asthma, heart block or acute heart failure

- **A**CEI: to reduce adverse cardiac remodelling and angiotensin-induced vasoconstriction
- **S**tatins: reduce cholesterol levels, improve endothelial function and maintain atherosclerotic plaque stability
- **H**eparin: LMWH e.g. dalteparin.

Although warfarin is a good anticoagulant, it is slower to act than dual antiplatelet therapy and it causes an initial prothrombotic phase when treatment is commenced. Therefore, it is not used in the acute management of an acute coronary syndrome.

25. A

This patient is describing a case of drug-induced gynaecomastia. Gynaecomastia is the presence of an abnormally large amount of breast tissue in men. It has many intrinsic causes such as hypogonadism, cirrhosis and oestrogen-producing tumours. Drug side-effects are also a common cause of gynaecomastia with the main culprits being: Oestrogens, spironolactone, digoxin and cimetidine. Cimetidine is a histamine receptor antagonist that is used to treat peptic ulcer disease and GORD. Although there is no mention of this patient having either of these diseases, cimetidine is the only option that is known to cause gynaecomastia.

26. B

Benign prostatic hyperplasia (BPH) refers to the slowly progressive nodular hyperplasia of the periurethral (transitional) zone of the prostate gland. BPH is the most common cause of lower urinary tract symptoms in adult males. The transitional zone surrounds the urethra as it enters the prostate gland. It is small in young adults and gradually grows throughout life. The peripheral zone contains most of the prostate's glandular tissue and around 80% of prostate cancer originates from this zone. The central zone is the area surrounding the ejaculatory ducts.

27. B

A cramping pain in lower limb muscle groups that occurs on exertion is consistent with intermittent claudication. This is caused by peripheral vascular disease leading to reduced blood flow to muscles of the lower limbs. Intermittent claudication of the buttocks occurs due to partial occlusion of the aorta at the point at which it becomes the iliac arteries (hence, it is sometimes called 'aortoiliac occlusive disease'). It also leads to erectile dysfunction and reduced/absent distal pulses — this constellation of signs and symptoms is known as Leriche Syndrome.

Intermittent claudication can progress to critical limb ischaemia as the peripheral vascular disease worsens. Critical limb ischaemia is characterised by rest pain, night pain (relieved by dangling the affected leg over the end of the bed) and tissue loss (gangrene and ulcers). Chronic compartment syndrome occurs when the pressure within a fascial compartment increases during exercise, causing pain. Spinal stenosis is caused by narrowing of the spinal canal, which applies pressure on the spinal cord. Lumbar spinal stenosis causes pain in the lower limbs when walking or standing for long periods of time. The pain is eased by bending forward (often mentioned in SBAs) or sitting down.

28. B

Behçet's disease is a systemic inflammatory disease of unknown cause that presents with a triad of mouth ulcers, genital ulcers and uveitis.

Inflammatory bowel disease has several extra-GI manifestations such as uveitis and oral ulcers but is not associated with causing genital ulcers. Herpes simplex virus can cause a range of diseases including pharyngitis, encephalitis, cold sores and genital rash. Syphilis is a sexually-transmitted bacterial infection caused by *Treponema pallidum*. It usually presents with a single painless genital ulcer. This is then followed by a widespread painless rash and lymphadenopathy. If the disease continues to worsen, patients may develop neurosyphilis, cardiovascular syphilis or gummatous syphilis (formation of soft balls of inflammatory tissue). Reactive arthritis occurs in patients who have recently recovered from an infection (e.g. *Campylobacter jejuni* infections or urogenital infections). It causes a clinical triad of arthritis, urethritis and uveitis (previously known as Reiter's syndrome).

29. D

The most common ECG finding in PE patients is sinus tachycardia. PE can also show evidence of right heart strain, such as right axis deviation and right bundle branch block (RBBB). In the long-term, PE can produce ECG features of right ventricular hypertrophy. S1Q3T3 refers to the presence of a deep S wave in lead I, pathological Q wave in lead III and an inverted T wave in lead III. It is regarded as being a 'classic' feature of PE and is often used in SBAs, but it actually occurs relatively infrequently.

Tall tented T waves is a feature of hyperkalaemia, along with flattened P waves, broad QRS complexes and bradycardia. Reverse tick sign is a feature of digoxin toxicity. T wave inversion can be an early sign of myocardial ischaemia, however, it can also be a normal ECG variant.

30. E

Parkinson's disease is a neurodegenerative disorder caused by the loss of dopaminergic neurons in the substantia nigra. The characteristic features of Parkinson's disease are pill-rolling resting tremor, lead pipe muscle rigidity, bradykinesia, narrow gait (which is stooped and shuffling with reduced arm swing) and postural instability. Other, subtler, features to be aware of include hypomimia (reduced facial expression), hypophonia (soft voice), micrographia (progressively smaller handwriting), drooling tendency and furrowed eyebrows. Psychiatric disturbances such as anxiety, depression and cognitive impairment are also common.

Paper 7

Questions

1. What is the most common inheritance pattern of polycystic kidney disease?

   A Autosomal dominant
   B Autosomal recessive
   C X-linked dominant
   D X-linked recessive
   E Mitochondrial

2. Which of the following statements about inflammatory bowel disease is false?

   A Crohn's disease causes transmural inflammation, whereas UC causes inflammation of the mucosa or submucosa
   B Crohn's disease causes skip lesions, whereas UC is continuous
   C Crohn's disease is associated with abscesses, fistulae, adhesions and strictures, whereas UC is associated with toxic megacolon
   D Crohn's disease favours the rectum, whereas UC favours the terminal ileum

    E Barium follow-through will show rose-thorn ulcers and a cobblestone mucosa in Crohn's disease, but a lead pipe mucosa in UC

3. A 68-year-old care home resident is brought into A&E hyperventilating and complaining of a 'ringing sound' in her ears. She has a low-grade fever and appears to be confused. She has a past medical history of depression and a TIA (2 months ago). What is the most likely diagnosis?

    A Aspirin overdose
    B Paracetamol overdose
    C TCA overdose
    D Cerebrovascular accident
    E Pneumonia

4. A 25-year-old male presents to his GP complaining of a lump in his armpit. He says it doesn't usually hurt except for when he goes out binge drinking with his friends. In the past few months, he has noticed that his clothes have become quite loose-fitting and he has been getting very hot and sweaty more than usual. On examination, he has firm, rubbery axillary lymphadenopathy, splenomegaly and scratch marks on his arms.

    A Multiple myeloma
    B Chronic lymphocytic leukaemia
    C Chronic myeloid leukaemia
    D Non-Hodgkin's lymphoma
    E Hodgkin's lymphoma

5. A 68-year-old man presents to his GP complaining of a cough that has been bothering him for 3 months. He says that he has coughed up large volumes of 'rusty-coloured' sputum. According to his hospital notes, he has been admitted 4 times in the past 12 months due to pneumonia. On examination, his fingers are clubbed and coarse crepitations are heard at the lung bases. What is the most likely underlying diagnosis?

   A COPD
   B Bronchiectasis
   C Pneumonia
   D Interstitial lung disease
   E TB

6. A 55-year-old woman is receiving treatment for chronic myeloid leukaemia. The consultant is concerned that this patient may have developed tumour lysis syndrome and requests some blood tests. What would you expect to see in the blood results of a patient with tumour lysis syndrome?

   A Low K^+, High PO_4^{3-}, High Ca^{2+} and High Uric Acid
   B High K^+, High PO_4^{3-}, Low Ca^{2+} and High Uric Acid
   C High K^+, Low Na^+, Low Ca^{2+} and High Mg^{2+}
   D Low K^+, High Na^+, Low Mg^{2+} and High Uric Acid
   E High Ca^{2+}, Low PO_4^{3-} and High Uric Acid

7. Which of the following is a cardiac cause of finger clubbing?

   A Congenital cyanotic heart disease
   B Viral pericarditis
   C Dilated cardiomyopathy
   D Rheumatic fever
   E Wolff–Parkinson–White syndrome

8. A 39-year-old homeless man is brought into A&E having been found lying in a pool of blood on the street. He is known to the A&E department having frequently been admitted for alcohol-related issues. There are no obvious signs of trauma and blood is seen in and around his mouth. Vital Signs: HR = 110 bpm; BP = 87/61 mmHg. On examination, splenomegaly, shifting dullness and dilated veins on the anterior abdomen are identified. The registrar suspects a variceal bleed secondary to portal hypertension. What is the first step in this patient's management?

    A TIPS procedure
    B Band ligation
    C Terlipressin and prophylactic antibiotics
    D Beta-blockers
    E Terlipressin and beta-blockers

9. A 23-year-old woman comes to see her GP about some breast lumps that she has noticed over the past 6 months. She mentions that her breasts become quite painful and feel 'lumpy', especially in the few days before her period. The pain is relieved when she has her period. What is the most likely diagnosis?

    A Fibrocystic disease
    B Fibroadenoma
    C Breast cancer
    D Breast abscess
    E Duct ectasia

10. A 92-year-old female, with a history of osteoporosis, is brought into A&E by her grandson. He says that she has been drifting in and out of consciousness for the past 2 weeks and has been complaining of a headache that has been keeping her up at night and getting progressively more severe. On examination, her left pupil is dilated and displaced downwards and outwards. What investigation should be performed first?

    A Lumbar puncture
    B Carotid artery Doppler
    C CT head
    D EEG
    E Transthoracic echocardiogram

11. A 29-year-old man presents with a 4-day history of high fever. On inspection, you notice some needle track marks on his arms and a pansystolic murmur is heard on auscultation, which had not

previously been documented in his hospital notes. What is the most likely diagnosis?

A Mitral regurgitation
B Pericarditis
C Infective endocarditis
D Aortic stenosis
E Mitral valve prolapse

12. Which of the following is not part of the criteria for diagnosing SLE?

A Pleurisy
B Thrombocytopaenia
C Anti-dsDNA antibodies
D Oral ulcers
E Heliotrope rash

13. A 43-year-old woman presents with a 2-month history of diarrhoea and weight loss. She has also been feeling anxious about her appearance, as many people have commented that she always looks like she is staring. On examination, her eyes appear slightly protruded and lid lag is demonstrated. She has a fine tremor in both her hands and a lumpy skin lesion is noticed on her shins. What is the most likely diagnosis?

A Toxic multinodular goitre
B Graves' disease
C De Quervain's thyroiditis
D Hashimoto's thyroiditis
E Riedel's thyroiditis

14. A 76-year-old man is admitted to hospital with a cough productive of green sputum. He has also experienced some shortness of breath and a fever. A week before his admission, his carers noted that he had a high fever, malaise and myalgia for a few days. A chest X-ray shows

a cavitating lesion with an air fluid level. What is the most likely causative organism?

    A *Staphylococcus aureus*
    B *Streptococcus pneumoniae*
    C *Legionella pneumophila*
    D *Mycoplasma pneumonia*
    E *Haemophilus influenzae*

15. The urine output of a 78-year-old inpatient on the surgical ward has decreased gradually over the past 24 hrs despite maintaining an adequate fluid intake. The nurses add that he has recently become rather confused and complains of nausea. U&Es are requested:

    Creatinine: 231 — mmol/L (baseline: 97)
    Urea: 12.5 mmol/L (2.5–6.7)
    Na^+: 139 mmol/L (135–145)
    K^+: 6.1 mmol/L (3.5–5)

An AKI is diagnosed. He is currently on ramipril (for his hypertension), bisoprolol (for his paroxysmal AF) and ibuprofen.

Which of the following steps is inappropriate in this patient's management?

    A Assess and optimise fluid status
    B 10 mL of 10% calcium gluconate IV
    C Stop ramipril
    D Stop bisoprolol
    E Stop ibuprofen

16. A 57-year-old man is complaining of numbness and weakness in his arms. It began in his hands, 2 weeks ago, but for the last 3 days his forearms have also felt numb. On examination, there is no sensation below his elbows, tone is reduced bilaterally and the biceps and

brachioradialis reflexes cannot be elicited. He adds that he recently recovered from a bout of diarrhoea and vomiting. What is the most likely diagnosis?

    A Multiple sclerosis
    B Motor neuron disease
    C Parkinson's disease
    D Guillain–Barré syndrome
    E Huntington's disease

17. A 77-year-old patient with cirrhosis presents to A&E with diffuse abdominal pain, abdominal heaviness and fever. Associated symptoms include nausea and vomiting. On examination, shifting dullness is demonstrated and a fluid thrill is observed. What investigation should form part of the initial diagnostic work-up?

    A Abdominal X-ray
    B Abdominal ultrasound
    C Abdominal CT
    D Diagnostic paracentesis
    E Stool sample for MC&S

18. Which of the following is the correct chronological sequence of retinal changes that occur in hypertensive retinopathy?

    A Papilloedema → Silver Wiring → Flame Haemorrhages → AV Nipping
    B Silver Wiring → AV Nipping → Flame Haemorrhages → Papilloedema
    C Silver Wiring → Flame Haemorrhages → AV Nipping → Papilloedema
    D AV Nipping → Papilloedema → Silver Wiring → Flame Haemorrhages
    E AV Nipping → Silver Wiring → Papilloedema → Flame Haemorrhages

19. A 44-year-old woman is complaining of pain and a tingling feeling in the lateral half of her right hand. She often finds that she wakes up in the middle of the night because of the pain, which is then relieved by shaking her hand vigorously. Which nerve has been affected?

    A Ulnar nerve
    B Radial nerve
    C Musculocutaneous nerve
    D Median nerve
    E Posterior interosseous nerve

20. Which of the following full blood count and clotting screen results is consistent with a diagnosis of disseminated intravascular coagulation?

    A High platelets, High Hb, High APTT/PT, High fibrinogen
    B High platelets, High Hb, Low APTT/PT, High fibrinogen
    C Low platelets, High Hb, Low APTT/PT, Low fibrinogen
    D Low platelets, Low Hb, High APTT/PT, Low fibrinogen
    E Low platelets, Low Hb, Low APTT/PT, Low fibrinogen

21. A 40-year-old woman is admitted to A&E with shortness of breath that began suddenly a day after she returned from a holiday to the Maldives. What is the first step in her management?

    A D-dimer
    B High flow oxygen and low molecular weight heparin
    C IV heparin
    D CTPA
    E Venous ultrasound of the lower limbs

22. What is the gold standard diagnostic test for acromegaly?

    A Insulin suppression test
    B Oral glucose tolerance test
    C Short synacthen test

D IGF-1 levels

E Thyroid function test

23. Which of the following sets of results would be consistent with alcoholic hepatitis?

    A Elevated MCV, ALT:AST > 2 and elevated GGT

    B Elevated MCV, AST:ALT > 2 and elevated GGT

    C Reduced MCV, AST:ALT > 2 and elevated GGT

    D Elevated MCV, ALT:AST > 2 and reduced GGT

    E Reduced MCV, AST:ALT > 2 and reduced GGT

24. An inpatient on the orthopaedic surgery ward has recently developed a cough, high fevers and chills. Blood cultures are taken which identify MRSA. Which of the following antibiotics is often used in the treatment of MRSA infections?

    A Vancomycin

    B Flucloxacillin

    C Tazocin

    D Metronidazole

    E Cefuroxime

25. A 77-year-old man is referred to the outpatient clinic by his GP having presented with chest pain and worsening shortness of breath. He has a history of COPD, diagnosed 12 years ago. On examination, his JVP is elevated, a parasternal heave is palpated and auscultation reveals an early diastolic murmur. An ECG is performed which shows right-axis deviation, a tall R wave in V1 and peaked P waves in lead ll. What is the most likely diagnosis?

    A Aortic regurgitation

    B Mitral stenosis

    C Pulmonary hypertension

    D Right heart failure

    E Exacerbation of COPD

26. Which of the following is not a histopathological type of malignant melanoma?

    A Superficial spreading
    B Acral lentiginous
    C Bowen's disease
    D Nodular
    E Lentigo maligna

27. An 82-year-old man has recently suffered from a right-sided stroke and is undergoing physiotherapy. He is referred for an upper limb neurological examination. The power in his right arm is normal. He can abduct his left arm by himself, but fails to maintain that position as soon as any resistance is applied. What is the MRC grading of his left shoulder abduction?

    A Grade 1
    B Grade 2
    C Grade 3
    D Grade 4
    E Grade 5

28. A 54-year-old female, with a BMI of 28, presents with a 2-year history of epigastric pain that radiates to the neck. It gets worse when lying down, and she also complains of painless regurgitation of food. What is the most appropriate investigation to confirm the diagnosis?

    A Chest X-ray
    B Barium swallow
    C ECG
    D OGD
    E Manometry

29. Which of the following is not an indication for dialysis in the context of acute kidney injury?

    A Refractory hyperkalaemia
    B Refractory pulmonary oedema

C Uraemic pericarditis
D Severe metabolic acidosis
E Macroscopic haematuria

30. A 25-year-old man, with no past medical history, presents to A&E with sudden-onset shortness of breath and right-sided chest pain, which started whilst he was playing football. Vital Signs: RR = 24/min; HR = 125 bpm; BP = 85/59 mm Hg. There is a hyper-resonant percussion note and reduced breath sounds over the right upper zone and the trachea is deviated to the left. A chest X-ray confirms the presence of a pneumothorax measuring 3 cm. What is the most appropriate management option?

A Give analgesia and reassure
B Admit to hospital, monitor vital signs and repeat chest X-ray in 3 hrs
C Insert a chest drain
D Insert a large-bore cannula into the right 2nd intercostal space in the midclavicular line
E Surgical pleurectomy

Answers

1. A

Inheritance patterns don't often come up in SBAs, however, you should be aware of the inheritance patterns of a few important conditions.

> **Autosomal Dominant** — Polycystic Kidney Disease (more rarely, PKD can be autosomal recessive), Hereditary Haemorrhagic Telangiectasia, Peutz–Jeghers syndrome, Huntingdon's disease, Marfan's syndrome, MEN syndrome
> **Autosomal Recessive** — Cystic Fibrosis, Sickle Cell Disease, Thalassemia
> **X-linked Recessive** — Red-Green Colour Blindness, Haemophilia, G6PD deficiency

2. D

Crohn's diseases and ulcerative colitis are related conditions that fall under the umbrella of 'inflammatory bowel disease'. They present in reasonably similar ways, however, there are some important differences that are often tested in SBAs. These differences are summarised in the table below:

	Ulcerative colitis	Crohn's disease
Presentation	Diffuse abdominal pain, PR blood and mucus	Right iliac fossa pain, failure to thrive between attacks
Examination	Clubbing, anterior uveitis, erythema nodosum, pyoderma gangrenosum, signs of anaemia	
		Aphthous ulcers, fissures and fistulae
Commonly affected location	Rectum	Terminal ileum
Distribution	Rectum and colon	Any point from mouth to anus
Pattern of inflammation	Continuous lesions	Skip lesions (discontinuous)
Depth of inflammation	Confined to mucosa or submucosa	Transmural

(*Continued*)

(Continued)

	Ulcerative colitis	Crohn's disease
Bile duct involvement	Increased risk of PSC	None
Smoking	Protective	Increases risk
Barium follow-through findings	Lead-pipe mucosa	Rose-thorn ulcers, cobblestone mucosa
Biopsy findings	Mucosal ulcers, goblet cell depletion and crypt abscesses	Non-caseating granuloma
Management	Remission maintained with topical or oral aminosalicylates (e.g. mesalazine)	Stop smoking, remission maintained with steroid-sparing agents (e.g. azathioprine)
Surgery	Potentially curative	Not curative, high rate of recurrence
Complications	Colonic adenocarcinoma, toxic megacolon	Abscesses, fistulae, adhesions, strictures, fissures, obstruction and perforation

3. A

Aspirin overdose usually presents with fever, sweating, hyperventilation and tinnitus or deafness. Important clues in this SBA include the past medical history of TIA, which would mean that she is likely to be on aspirin for secondary prevention, and depression, as most cases of aspirin overdose are due to attempted suicide or self-harm. Aspirin is an acid (acetylsalicylic acid), so overdose causes metabolic acidosis. The mainstay of treatment is alkaline diuresis with IV sodium bicarbonate.

Paracetamol overdose is usually asymptomatic for the first 24 hrs and then presents with features of liver failure (such as confusion, jaundice and vomiting). Tricyclic anti-depressant overdose typically presents with tachycardia, drowsiness, dry mouth, nausea/vomiting and confusion. The hyperventilation and low-grade fever may bring pneumonia into consideration, however, it would not cause tinnitus and is likely to present with a cough.

4. E

Painless lymphadenopathy (axillary in this case) that becomes painful after ingestion of alcohol is pathognomonic of Hodgkin's lymphoma. The lymph nodes are often described as being 'firm and rubbery'. A lymphoma is a neoplasm of lymphoid tissue usually arising in the lymph nodes. Hodgkin's lymphoma is a histopathological diagnosis based on the presence of Reed–Sternberg cells in a lymph node biopsy. They are giant cells derived from B lymphocytes containing two or more oval nuclei with eosinophilic nucleoli resembling 'owl eyes'. Epstein–Barr Virus (EBV) is implicated in up to 50% of cases of Hodgkin's lymphoma. This patient is also experiencing the B symptoms of lymphoma: fever >38°C (known as Pel-Ebstein fever if cyclical), unintentional weight loss and night sweats. The presence of B symptoms is associated with a poor prognosis. Other symptoms include pruritus (hence, the scratch marks seen on this patient), a persistent cough and back pain. Splenomegaly is a common examination finding present in approximately 30% of patients.

5. B

A cough productive of large volumes of purulent sputum (which can become 'rusty-coloured' during infections) and recurrent respiratory infections are features of bronchiectasis. It is characterised by chronic dilation of the bronchi, impaired clearance of mucus and, consequentially, recurrent respiratory tract infections. Other symptoms include haemoptysis, dyspnoea, chest pain and weight loss. Examination findings may include clubbing (rare), coarse crepitations and a wheeze.

COPD is more likely to present with worsening shortness of breath and a cough productive of clear sputum (although infections are also common). Furthermore, COPD is not associated with clubbing. Although this could, in theory, be a new episode of community-acquired pneumonia, the history of several pneumonias over the past year and the presence of clubbing are suggestive of an underlying disease process, such as bronchiectasis. Interstitial lung disease causes fine crepitations and is classically associated with occupational exposure to organic or mineral dusts. TB is usually quite easy to recognise in SBAs as it will classically present in patients who are originally from, or have recently travelled to, a TB-endemic country complaining of dyspnoea, haemoptysis and weight loss (with associated extra-pulmonary manifestations such as painless lymphadenopathy, lupus vulgaris and erythema nodusum).

6. B

Tumour lysis syndrome (TLS) is a group of metabolic abnormalities that results from cancer treatment. Cytotoxic drugs lead to the lysis of large numbers of cancer cells, which release their contents into the bloodstream. TLS most commonly occurs in the treatment of leukaemia and lymphoma. The main metabolic derangements in TLS are: High K^+, High PO_4^{3-}, High Uric Acid and Low Ca^{2+}.

7. A

The cardiac causes of finger clubbing are congenital cyanotic heart disease (most common), atrial myxoma (benign tumour of the heart), subacute bacterial endocarditis and tetralogy of Fallot (a combination of four congenital heart defects: ventricular septal defect, pulmonary stenosis, right ventricular hypertrophy and an overriding aorta).

8. C

Oesophageal varices are dilated sub-mucosal collateral veins found in the lower ⅓ of the oesophagus that arise due to portal hypertension. A high portal pressure results in blood being shunted into areas of lower venous pressure such as sites of portosystemic anastomosis. When the portal pressure is >12 mm Hg, these anastomoses become congested and dilated, and are prone to bleeding. Portal hypertension can be remembered as causing problems in the 'butt' (haemorrhoids), 'gut' (oesophageal varices) and 'caput' (caput medusae) as these are the sites of portosystemic anastomosis. The causes of portal hypertension can be divided into pre-hepatic (e.g. portal vein thrombosis), hepatic (e.g. cirrhosis, schistosomiasis) and post-hepatic (e.g. Budd–Chiari syndrome, right heart failure, constrictive pericarditis).

As soon as a variceal bleed is suspected, Terlipressin should be administered — this is a vasopressin analogue that causes splanchnic vasoconstriction, thereby reducing mesenteric blood flow and portal pressure. Short-term prophylactic antibiotics should also be administered as this reduces the risk of infection, re-bleeding and mortality. Endoscopy should be performed within 12 hrs of the onset of bleeding to diagnose and treat variceal haemorrhage, either with band ligation or injection sclerotherapy. If the combined pharmacological and endoscopic treatment fails, a transjugular intrahepatic portosystemic shunt (TIPS) may be considered. This is a surgical intervention that reduces portal hypertension. Non-selective beta-blockade is used to prevent variceal bleeds in patients at high risk.

9. A

Fibrocystic disease is a very common benign breast condition characterised by lumpy breasts which can be painful. The pain is typically at its worst immediately before the patient's period and is relieved when the period arrives.

A fibroadenoma is a discrete breast lump that is firm, smooth and mobile. They are sometimes referred to as 'breast mice'. The presence of multiple lumps makes this diagnosis unlikely. Breast cancer tends to cause an irregular, firm lump that appears attached to surrounding breast tissue. There may also be a bloody nipple discharge and axillary lymphadenopathy. Other specific signs of breast cancer include Paget's disease of the breast and peau d'orange. Breast abscess will present with a painful and tender breast showing the classic signs of inflammation (red, hot, swollen, etc.). The patient is also likely to be systemically unwell with a fever. It is most common in women who are breastfeeding, and smoking is a major risk factor. Duct ectasia is a condition in which the lactiferous ducts get blocked. The classic SBA buzzword of duct ectasia is a *'cheesy yellow/ green discharge'*.

10. C

To summarise, the key features of this patient's history are fluctuating consciousness, a gradually worsening headache that is worst when lying down (thus disturbing her sleep) and oculomotor nerve palsy (down and out pupil). The features of raised ICP (e.g. a headache that is worst when lying down) allude to a space-occupying lesion compressing surrounding structures, such as the oculomotor nerve, as the underlying cause of this patient's condition. Fluctuating consciousness is a typical feature of subdural haematoma, in which blood accumulates in between the dura mater and arachnoid mater. The patient is elderly and frail, meaning that she is at high risk of falls. It is likely that she has fallen and sustained some degree of head trauma (although not explicitly mentioned), which has led to her current condition. Subdural haematomas are classified based on the speed of onset of symptoms: acute <72 hrs; subacute — 3–20 days; chronic >3 weeks. The diagnosis is confirmed using a CT head scan which will show a sickle or crescent-shaped mass. Lumbar puncture is contraindicated in these patients as the raised ICP can lead to brainstem herniation. Transthoracic echocardiogram and carotid artery Doppler scans are used to investigate sources of emboli in patients who have suffered a stroke/TIA. EEG aids the diagnosis of epilepsy.

11. C

This SBA is designed to catch you out. Heart murmurs are taught quite extensively in the first clinical year of medical school so buzzwords such as 'pansystolic murmur' will make many students jump to a diagnosis of mitral regurgitation without considering the rest of the clinical picture. It is true that mitral regurgitation and ventricular septal defect can cause a pansystolic murmur, however, the signs of IV drug use (needle track marks), fever and new-onset murmur paints a typical picture of infective endocarditis. IV drug use is a major risk factor for infective endocarditis as non-sterile techniques can lead to the introduction of *S. aureus* into the circulation. Another risk factor that is commonly seen in SBAs is recent dental surgery which can result in *S. viridans* bacteraemia. Bacterial vegetations typically grow on the tricuspid valve and are most often associated with tricuspid regurgitation (which also causes a pansystolic murmur).

Pericarditis causes a pericardial friction rub on auscultation. Aortic stenosis causes an ejection systolic murmur. Mitral valve prolapse causes a mid-systolic click and an end-systolic murmur (also known as a Barlow murmur).

12. E

Systemic lupus erythematosus (SLE) is a multisystem autoimmune disease in which the immune system produces antibodies against a variety of self-antigens, resulting in widespread tissue damage. As SLE has a diverse range of manifestations, it can often masquerade as other illnesses. To assist with the diagnosis of SLE, the revised criteria was produced. SLE can be diagnosed if 4 or more of the following 11 features are present:

> **S**erositis (pleuritis, pericarditis)
> **O**ral ulcer
> **A**rthritis (non-erosive)
> **P**hotosensitivity
> **B**lood disorders (haemolytic anaemia, leukopaenia, thrombocytopaenia)
> **R**enal disorders (e.g. proteinuria, red cell casts)
> **A**nti-nuclear antibodies (ANA)
> **I**mmunological disorders (presence of anti-dsDNA/anti-Sm/ anti-phospholipid antibodies)
> **N**eurological disease (psychosis, seizures)
> **M**alar rash (butterfly rash)
> **D**iscoid rash
> Mnemonic: **SOAP BRAIN MD**

13. B

Unintentional weight loss, diarrhoea and anxiety are features of all forms of hyperthyroidism. Exophthalmos and pretibial myxedema ('a lumpy skin lesion'), on the other hand, are specific to Graves' disease. They are associated with the presence of TSH-receptor stimulating antibodies.

Hashimoto's thyroiditis causes hypothyroidism. Riedel's thyroiditis is a condition in which normal thyroid tissue is replaced by dense fibrous tissue. The thyroid becomes very hard, and is sometimes described in SBAs as being 'woody'. Most patients with Riedel's thyroiditis will be euthyroid, and about 30% will become hypothyroid.

14. A

This patient has presented with features of pneumonia: cough, fever and shortness of breath. The most common cause of community-acquired pneumonia is *Streptococcus pneumoniae* but this does not tend to cause a cavitating lesion with an air-fluid level. Infectious causes of cavitating lesions include *Staphylococcus aureus*, *Klebsiella pneumoniae* and TB. Other causes include squamous cell carcinoma of the lung, rheumatoid arthritis and granulomatosis with polyangiitis (previously known as Wegener's granulomatosis). *S. aureus* tends to cause a post-influenza pneumonia. A preceding influenza infection will cause sufficient damage to the respiratory system such that *S. aureus* can then infect. Therefore, the combination of systemic symptoms of pneumonia, a cavitating lesion with an air-fluid level and a preceding flu-like illness, makes **option A** most likely.

Legionella pneumophila and *Mycoplasma pneumonia* are causes of atypical pneumonia. Atypical pneumonia causes vague symptoms such as fever, malaise, myalgia followed by a dry cough. Each cause of atypical pneumonia has distinctive associations, such as *Legionella* and air conditioning units (more on this later). *Haemophilus influenzae* is another common cause of community-acquired pneumonia.

15. D

The general management of AKI can be divided into four main components: Protecting from hyperkalaemia, optimising fluid balance, stopping nephrotoxic drugs and assessing the need for dialysis. Hyperkalaemia is a dangerous consequence of AKI as it can lead to fatal arrhythmias. To protect against this, 10 mL 10% calcium gluconate IV should be given. It is cardioprotective, however, it does not affect serum potassium levels. IV insulin and dextrose is required to lower serum potassium. Other options include salbutamol nebulizers and IV sodium bicarbonate. The patient's ECG should be monitored for signs of improvement. AKI patients may be dehydrated or fluid overloaded, so it is important to assess fluid status by looking at key signs such as JVP, tissue turgor, blood pressure and pulse rate. Fluids should be titrated to maintain fluid balance. Nephrotoxic drugs can cause or worsen AKI so they should be stopped immediately. Common examples of nephrotoxic drugs include ACE inhibitors, NSAIDs, gentamicin and amphotericin. Beta-blockers are not nephrotoxic and do not need to be stopped acutely. The need for dialysis is based on the severity of the complications of AKI.

16. D

Guillain–Barré syndrome (GBS) is an acute inflammatory demyelinating polyneuropathy that causes hypotonia, flaccid paralysis, arreflexia, impairment of sensation and bulbar palsy. It is characterised by progressive ascending symmetrical limb weakness and numbness, as seen in this patient. Most patients with GBS will have recently suffered from a respiratory or gastrointestinal infection (most often caused by *C. jejuni*). Some patients will develop respiratory muscle weakness, which can lead to respiratory failure. GBS tends to be a relatively acute disease with a history spanning a matter of weeks.

Motor neuron disease causes symptoms and signs of upper and/or lower motor neuron lesions. It does not cause sensory impairment. Multiple sclerosis is also an inflammatory demyelinating disease of the nervous system; however, it is usually diagnosed by the presence of two episodes of neurological symptoms separated in time and space (i.e. location of the lesion). Although it can present acutely (particularly the Marburg variant of MS), the mention of a recent diarrhoeal illness makes GBS more likely. Parkinson's disease is characterised by bradykinesia, postural instability, rigidity and a resting 'pill-rolling' tremor. Huntington's disease is an autosomal dominant neurological condition typically presenting with behavioural and psychiatric changes and jerky movements (chorea).

17. D

Patients with cirrhosis are at a particularly high risk of spontaneous bacterial peritonitis (SBP). This is an acute bacterial infection of the ascitic fluid, which has no obvious source. The bacteria most commonly involved are *E. coli* and *Klebsiella pneumoniae*. In any patient with a history of liver disease presenting with ascites and a fever, SBP needs to be excluded via diagnostic paracentesis. A peritoneal fluid neutrophil count >250 cells/mm^3 is diagnostic of SBP.

18. B

This is known as the Keith–Wagener classification of hypertensive retinopathy:

Grade 1 = Silver Wiring
Grade 2 = AV Nipping
Grade 3 = Flame Haemorrhages and Cotton Wool Exudates
Grade 4 = Papilloedema

19. D

Carpal tunnel syndrome refers to a constellation of symptoms caused by compression of the median nerve as it runs through the carpal tunnel. It leads to sensory impairment in the distribution of the median nerve (lateral half of the palm and the first three digits) leading to a tingling pain and weakness of the affected hand. Carpal tunnel syndrome is usually idiopathic but obesity, infiltrative diseases and fluid-retention states (e.g. pregnancy) can increase risk.

20. D

Disseminated intravascular coagulation (DIC) is characterised by widespread activation of the clotting cascade resulting in depletion of clotting factors and platelets. DIC has many causes including Gram-negative sepsis, severe pre-eclampsia and acute promyelocytic leukaemia. The cascade, that leads to DIC, stems from endothelial injury resulting in the release of procoagulant substances and, subsequently, activation of the clotting cascade. Microangiopathic haemolytic anaemia is a component of DIC, and it is responsible for the low Hb seen in DIC patients. The consumption of clotting factors and platelets leads to a low platelet count and prolonged clotting times.

21. B

This is a typical case of pulmonary embolism. The main causes of sudden-onset shortness of breath in relatively young people are pulmonary embolism, pneumothorax, anaphylaxis and asthma attack. Often, SBAs will mention a key risk factor for DVT/PE such as long-haul travel, recent surgery or the oral contraceptive pill.

The immediate management of PE involves delivering high-flow oxygen and subcutaneous LMWH (e.g. enoxaparin). Once this measure has been taken, a Wells score can be calculated and, dependent on the score, appropriate investigations (either a CTPA or D-dimer) can be performed. Venous ultrasound of the lower limbs is used to confirm the presence of a DVT.

22. B

Acromegaly is caused by high growth hormone (GH) levels in adults, most commonly caused by a GH-secreting pituitary adenoma. Aside from promoting anabolic activities within cells, GH also has an important role in increasing blood glucose levels. Therefore, it responds to blood glucose via a feedback loop (i.e. GH decreases when blood glucose increases). An oral glucose tolerance test temporarily raises blood glucose and the GH response is observed. Failure to suppress GH release using an oral glucose tolerance test is suggestive of acromegaly.

GH stimulates the production of IGF-1 (insulin-like growth factor) in the liver, which has several growth-stimulating effects in various tissues. Measuring the IGF-1 level is a useful screening tool in acromegaly as it is very sensitive, however, it lacks specificity so cannot be used, by itself, to confirm the diagnosis. Insulin suppression tests are used to investigate hypopituitarism.

23. B

Elevated MCV is common in alcoholic patients and occurs due to the harmful effect of alcohol on erythroblast development. The transaminases (ALT and AST) are usually found within hepatocytes, however, abnormal membrane permeability induced by alcohol leads to the leakage of these enzymes into the blood. This results in high serum transaminase levels. An AST to ALT ratio (AST:ALT) >2 is suggestive of liver damage secondary to alcohol abuse. Chronic alcohol consumption also induces a rise in serum GGT.

24. A

Methicillin-resistant *Staphylococcus aureus* (MRSA) is a hospital-acquired infection that may cause pneumonia, wound infections and septicaemia. It is extremely dangerous because of its drug-resistance. It is often treated with vancomycin.

Tazocin, a combination of tazobactam and piperacillin, is regularly used to treat hospital-acquired pneumonias. Cefuroxime is a cephalosporin antibiotic that is active against *H. influenzae* and *N. gonorrhoeae*.

25. C

A good point to start with in this question is the examination findings — in particular, the raised JVP. The three main causes of a raised JVP are constrictive pericarditis, right heart failure (secondary to left heart failure or pulmonary hypertension) and tricuspid regurgitation. This therefore narrows down the answer to either pulmonary hypertension or right heart failure. The parasternal heave and ECG findings (right axis deviation and tall R wave in V1) confirms the presence of right ventricular hypertrophy. The right ventricle undergoes hypertrophy when it has to pump against greater resistance, for example, in pulmonary hypertension. This patient also has an early diastolic murmur, present in aortic and pulmonary regurgitation. Aortic regurgitation is unlikely as the examination and ECG findings are consistent with a right-sided heart problem. This murmur is therefore due to pulmonary regurgitation (because of pulmonary hypertension) and is known as a Graham-Steell murmur.

Pulmonary hypertension is consistently elevated pulmonary arterial pressure (>20 mm Hg). It is either primary (idiopathic) or secondary to left heart disease, chronic lung disease (as in this patient), recurrent pulmonary emboli, increased pulmonary blood flow or connective tissue disease. Damaged lung tissue will not be able to fully saturate pulmonary arterial blood, which leads to pulmonary vasoconstriction in an attempt to divert the blood towards better oxygenating areas of lung tissue. Widespread pulmonary arterial vasoconstriction in patients with diffuse lung disease (e.g. COPD) leads to pulmonary hypertension. The peaked P wave on ECG is known as 'P pulmonale' and it signifies right atrial enlargement — a consequence of the right side of the heart having to pump against a greater resistance. Strictly speaking, this patient has cor pulmonale — defined as right heart failure resulting from a primary disorder of the lungs.

26. C

A melanoma is a neoplasm of melanocytes and there are four histopathological subtypes. The most common is superficial spreading melanoma — these tend to arise from a pre-existing naevus and are often described as a slowly changing mole. The earliest change tends to be an area of darkening with the lesion expanding radially rather than vertically. The second most common is nodular melanoma which tend to grow rapidly out of an area of skin with no pre-existing naevi (*de novo*). Nodular melanomas grow vertically as blue-black or blue-red nodules. Acral lentiginous melanomas are restricted to the soles of the feet and palms of the hands. It usually appears as a brown-black flat macule with irregular borders. Lentigo maligna melanoma is the least common subtype, arising from lentigo maligna (melanoma *in situ*) usually on sun-exposed skin. These are large, dark and can be nodular.

Bowen's disease is squamous cell carcinoma *in situ* (restricted to the epidermis). This is a pre-malignant condition and appears as a red-brown scaly patch most commonly on the arms, legs or trunk.

27. C

The Medical Research Council (MRC) scale is used in upper and lower limb neurological examinations to quantify muscle power. MRC Scale:

    Grade 0 = no muscle movement
    Grade 1 = flicker of movement
    Grade 2 = active movement with gravity eliminated
    Grade 3 = active movement against gravity (but not against
              resistance)
    Grade 4 = active movement against gravity and resistance
    Grade 5 = normal power

28. B

Symptomatic GORD (e.g. heartburn, belching, waterbrash), lower dysphagia and painless regurgitation of food, is the classic presentation of a hiatus hernia. This is when part of the stomach moves into the thoracic cavity via the diaphragmatic hiatus. There are two types: **Sliding** (gastro-oesophageal junction (GEJ) slides into the thorax) and **Rolling** (GEJ remains in place but a bulge of fundus herniates into the chest alongside the oesophagus). Around 80% of cases are sliding hiatus hernias. Barium swallow is the best investigation to confirm the diagnosis.

If the hiatus hernia is very large, a CXR may show a retrocardiac mass with an air-fluid level. An OGD, although useful for assessing damage to the oesophageal mucosa (e.g. Barrett's oesophagus) caused by GORD, cannot reliably exclude hiatus hernia. Manometry is used to measure lower oesophageal sphincter pressure and diagnose motility disorders. An ECG may be appropriate if a cardiac cause of the pain is suspected. Management of a hiatus hernia comprises of lifestyle changes (e.g. weight loss), treatment of reflux (PPIs) and surgery in refractory cases. Nissen fundoplication is the most commonly used surgical procedure for hiatus hernias.

29. E

Acute kidney injury (AKI) is an abrupt loss of kidney function resulting in the dysregulation of fluid balance and electrolytes, and the retention of nitrogenous waste products. The KDIGO criteria states that the diagnosis of an AKI requires:

- Rise in urea > 26 μmol/L in in 48 hrs
- Rise in creatinine > 1.5 × baseline (baseline measured in the last 3 months)
- Urine output < 0.5 mL/kg/h for > 6 hrs (i.e. your urine production in mL over 2 hrs should match your body weight in kg)

The indications for dialysis in AKI are:

- Refractory pulmonary oedema
- Persistent hyperkalaemia
- Severe metabolic acidosis

- Uraemic complications (e.g. encephalopathy, pericarditis)
- Drug overdose by the **BLAST** drugs: Barbiturates, Lithium, Alcohol, Salicylates and Theophyline

30. D

This young man has presented with a primary spontaneous pneumothorax. The patient is in shock (shown by the very low blood pressure) and his trachea is deviated, suggesting that this is a tension pneumothorax. In this condition, the lesion in the visceral pleura forms a one-way valve leading to the progressive accumulation of air in the pleural space, which requires urgent decompression. In this patient, decompression should be achieved by inserting a large-bore cannula into the right 2nd intercostal space in the mid-clavicular line. The patient should then be given high-flow oxygen and analgesia. Chest X-rays should be repeated to confirm the resolution of the pneumothorax. If left untreated, the gradually increasing volume of air within the pleural space can obstruct venous return to the heart, resulting in haemodynamic instability and cardiac arrest. Although tension pneumothorax patients in SBAs may present with several distinctive clinical features, in reality, most patients may only present with tachycardia, tachypnoea and hypoxia.

Management of spontaneous pneumothorax depends on the size and whether it is primary or secondary (occurring in patients with underlying lung disease).

Primary Pneumothorax
- <2 cm — reassurance, analgesia and discharge
- >2 cm — aspiration (discharge if successful, insert chest drain and administer high-flow oxygen if unsuccessful).

Secondary Pneumothorax
- <2 cm — aspiration (insert chest drain if unsuccessful)
- >2 cm — insert chest drain
- All secondary pneumothoraces require hospital admission and all patients should be given high-flow oxygen.

All pneumothoraces require a follow-up chest X-ray to confirm complete resolution. Surgical pleurectomy is the removal of the pleura, which may be considered in patients who suffer from recurrent pneumothoraces.

Paper 8

Questions

1. Which of the following organisms is a recognised cause of hospital-acquired pneumonia?

    A *Streptococcus pneumoniae*
    B *Pseudomonas aeruginosa*
    C *Haemophilus influenzae*
    D *Legionella pneumophila*
    E *Chlamydophila psittaci*

2. A 19-year-old girl visits her GP after experiencing painful urination over the past week. She has also been urinating more frequently than usual and complains that her urine looks cloudy and smells particularly bad. A urinary tract infection is suspected. Which investigation can definitively confirm the diagnosis?

    A Urine dipstick
    B CRP
    C Blood cultures
    D MSU
    E U&Es

3. A 31-year-old man presents with a 2-day history of diffuse watery diarrhoea and nausea. He admits to recently eating a BBQ at a friend's house. How should this patient be managed?

    A Bed rest and oral rehydration
    B Bed rest, oral rehydration and antibiotics
    C Anti-diarrhoeal agents
    D Call an ambulance and admit to hospital
    E Refer to a gastroenterologist for further investigation

4. A 16-year-old boy presents to his GP after noticing the growth of several small, fleshy tags on his torso. He has also noticed that he has many more 'birthmarks' now compared to when he was younger. On examination, there are eight coffee-coloured, flat skin lesions ('birthmarks') which are about 2–3 cm in diameter. Freckling around both axillae is also noted. What is the most likely diagnosis?

    A Tuberous sclerosis
    B Neurofibromatosis type 1
    C Neurofibromatosis type 2
    D Xeroderma pigmentosum
    E Dercum disease

5. Which of the following is an extra-articular feature of ankylosing spondylitis?

    A Erythema ab igne
    B Subcutaneous nodules
    C Apical lung fibrosis
    D Mitral regurgitation
    E Tophi

6. A 43-year-old man has been involved in a bar fight. He is rushed, unconscious, into A&E with a stab wound to the chest. On examination, his JVP is raised and he is hypotensive (BP: 86/70 mm Hg). Auscultation of his chest reveals very quiet heart sounds. What is the most likely diagnosis?

A Acute heart failure
B Haemopericardium
C Pneumothorax
D Septic shock
E Hypovolaemic shock

7. A 52-year-old man attends the respiratory clinic complaining of a dry
cough that has been bothering him for 2 months. He has never smoked
and has not experienced any shortness of breath or chest pain.
Respiratory examination detects no abnormalities. He has a past
medical history of hypertension, for which he started treatment 4
months ago. What is the most likely diagnosis?

A Asthma
B Interstitial lung disease
C Bronchiectasis
D Drug side-effect
E Atypical pneumonia

8. A 41-year-old female is referred to the dermatology clinic because
she has developed multiple purple nodules on her shins. They are
tender and have a diameter of 1–2 inches. Erythema nodusum is suspected. Which of the following is not a cause of erythema nodusum?

A Tuberculosis
B Reaction to sulphonamides
C Inflammatory bowel disease
D Ankylosing spondylitis
E Behçet's disease

9. A 49-year-old woman is admitted to A&E complaining of severe right
upper quadrant pain that began last evening and has not subsided. She
admits to eating a lot of fast food and mentions that, in the past, she
has experienced a stabbing pain for a couple of hours after eating. The
pain during these episodes is less intense than the pain she is currently
experiencing, and it tends to be localised around her epigastrium. She

drinks no more than 12 units of alcohol per week and has not lost any weight recently. On examination, she is jaundiced and Murphy's sign is positive. LFTs are requested:

Bilirubin: 45 μmol/L (3–17)
AST: 50 iU/L (5–35)
ALT: 45 iU/L (5–35)
ALP: 400 iU/L (30–150)

What is the most likely diagnosis?

A Gallstones
B Alcoholic hepatitis
C Viral hepatitis
D Hepatocellular carcinoma
E Gilbert's syndrome

10. A 34-year-old Nigerian man brings his 3-year-old son to A&E. He has been crying and complaining of severe pain in his hands. On examination, his fingers are swollen and warm. The junior doctor suspects a painful crises of sickle cell disease. What is the mode of inheritance of sickle cell disease?

A Autosomal recessive
B Autosomal dominant
C X-linked recessive
D X-linked dominant
E Y-linked

11. A 16-year-old girl is rushed to A&E by her parents. She is unconscious and shaking uncontrollably. Her mother says that she has been fitting for over half an hour. What is the most appropriate first step in the management of this patient?

A IV phenytoin
B IV thiopentone
C IV lorazepam/PR diazepam

D Reassure her parents and let the seizure terminate by itself

E Oral sodium valproate

12. A 61-year-old, with a 40 pack-year smoking history, presents with confusion. He has also had a 3-month history of weight loss and haemoptysis. A blood test shows the following results:

Na$^+$: 121 mmol/L (135–145)
K$^+$: 4.1 mmol/L (3.5–5)
Ca^{2+}: 2.3 mmol/L (2.2–2.6)

What is the most likely diagnosis?

A Addison's disease

B Hypothyroidism

C Heart failure

D SIADH

E Cirrhosis

13. A 27-year-old man presents complaining of sharp chest pain. He mentions that he has taken a few days off work recently because of the flu. What would you expect to see on his ECG?

A ST elevation in leads II, III, and aVF

B Widespread saddle-shaped ST elevation

C ST depression

D Tented T waves

E Absent P waves

14. Why are urinary tract infections more common in women?

A Women have a shorter urethra

B Men have a larger bladder

C Men have a shorter distance between their urethral opening and their anus

D Women are more likely to be catheterised

E Men have longer ureters

15. A 44-year-old bus driver from the West Indies has suffered from short-ness of breath and a dry cough for the last 4 months. He also com-plains of some 'sore lumps on his shins'. Closer inspection reveals tender violet nodules on both shins. A chest X-ray is requested, which shows bilateral hilar lymphadenopathy. Blood tests are also requested, including U&Es — which parameter would you expect to be raised?

> **A** Sodium
> **B** Potassium
> **C** Calcium
> **D** pH
> **E** Urea

16. A 35-year-old woman presents to clinic with a 6-month history of watery diarrhoea and abdominal pain that improves after defecation. She admits to defecating 4–5 times per day compared to her normal frequency of once per day. On examination, a papulovesicular rash is seen on both elbows. Which investigation would be most useful in aiding the diagnosis?

> **A** Stool sample for MC&S
> **B** Serology for anti-tTG antibodies
> **C** Full blood count
> **D** Blood cultures
> **E** Barium follow-through

17. Which of the following is a risk factor for breast cancer?

> **A** Breastfeeding
> **B** Late menarche
> **C** Early menopause
> **D** Not having children
> **E** Age <50 years

18. A 26-year-old man presents with an acutely swollen left knee. The pain and swelling started 2 days ago, but he didn't pay much attention

to it as he thought it was just a muscle strain. He has also developed a fever over the past 24 hrs. On examination, his left knee is red, swollen and extremely painful on passive flexion. Septic arthritis is suspected and a joint aspirate is requested. Which of the following organisms most commonly causes this condition?

    A *Haemophilus influenza*
    B *Staphylococcus aureus*
    C *Neisseria meningitidis*
    D *Escherichia coli*
    E *Mycobacterium tuberculosis*

19. A 44-year-old female presents to her GP complaining of worsening hearing. A full cranial nerves examination is performed. When Weber's test is performed, she hears the sound louder in her left ear. Then, Rinne's test is performed and she reports that, in both ears, the sound is loudest when the tuning fork is held in front of the auditory canal rather than when the fork is held against her mastoid processes. Which of the following best describes the patient's condition?

    A Conductive hearing loss in the right ear
    B Conductive hearing loss in the left ear
    C Sensorineural hearing loss in the right ear
    D Sensorineural hearing loss in the left ear
    E Bilateral sensorineural hearing loss

20. Which of the following best defines chronic kidney disease?

    A GFR < 60 mL/min/1.73m^2 for more than 3 months
    B GFR < 60 mL/min/1.73m^2 for more than 6 months
    C GFR < 90 mL/min/1.73m^2 for more than 3 months
    D GFR < 90 mL/min/1.73m^2 for more than 6 months
    E Requirement of long-term renal replacement therapy

21. A 77-year-old man, with a history of ischaemic heart disease, presents to A&E with acute-onset dyspnoea, a wheeze and a cough productive

of pink frothy sputum. A diagnosis of acute left ventricular failure, resulting in pulmonary oedema, is made. Which of the following is not part of the immediate management of this patient?

    A Administer oxygen
    B Lie the patient down
    C IV Diamorphine
    D GTN infusion
    E IV furosemide

22. Which of the following is not a cause of macrocytic anaemia?

    A Iron deficiency
    B Vitamin B12 deficiency
    C Folate deficiency
    D Methotrexate
    E Hypothyroidism

23. A 62-year-old shop owner is brought to A&E, by his daughter, having experienced worsening shortness of breath. His face and arms have also become quite swollen. On examination, he has a plethoric face and his JVP is raised and non-pulsatile. He seems disinterested when the history is taken because he does not trust doctors. His daughter adds that he has been coughing up blood and losing weight for about 6 months, however, he has refused to seek medical attention until his recent worsening of symptoms. What is the most likely diagnosis?

    A Asbestosis
    B Congestive cardiac failure
    C Polycythaemia
    D Superior vena cava syndrome
    E Mesothelioma

24. An 82-year-old man is brought to A&E with a severe headache. He complains of an intense aching pain, focused around his right eye

that has rapidly worsened. He has never experienced anything like this before. A nurse informs you that he vomited whilst waiting to be admitted, and has been complaining of nausea since. Closer inspection reveals a red, congested right eye with a cloudy cornea. He complains that his vision has worsened with the onset of this headache and he has started seeing haloes around all sources of light. What is the most likely diagnosis?

   A Meningitis
   B Subarachnoid haemorrhage
   C Acute glaucoma
   D Cluster headache
   E Migraine

25. Which of the following is associated with left ventricular systolic failure?

   A Pulsus alternans
   B Pulsus paradoxus
   C Water-hammer pulse
   D Pulsus parvus et tardus
   E Pulsus bisferiens

26. A 46-year-old truck driver is accompanied by his wife to see his GP after he fell asleep at the wheel two days ago. He appears to be quite shaken by the ordeal as he recalled having to veer away from oncoming traffic. On further questioning, he says that his sleep hasn't been disrupted, however, he has been feeling very tired during the day. His wife interjects and mentions that her own sleep has been disturbed because her husband has been 'snoring ferociously'. When asked about diet and exercise, he admits to eating badly and exercising very little since he started working as a truck driver 3 years ago. In that time, he has gained a considerable amount of weight. What is the most likely diagnosis?

    A Narcolepsy
    B Cataplexy
    C Absence seizure
    D Obstructive sleep apnoea
    E Central sleep apnoea

27. A 28-year-old IV drug-user visits his GP practice for an annual check-up. Hepatitis serology is requested and the following results are reported.

    HBsAg −
    HBeAg −
    HBcAb IgM −
    HBcAb IgG +
    HBsAb +

What is the hepatitis status of this patient?

    A Acute infection
    B Chronic infection
    C Cleared
    D Vaccinated
    E Susceptible

28. A 24-year-old student presents at his GP practice with a 2-day history of blood in his urine. Urine dipstick reveals proteinuria and haematuria. On questioning, he mentions that he has been recovering from a sore throat and a cough over the last 4 days. What is the most likely diagnosis?

    A Minimal change disease
    B IgA nephropathy
    C Membranous nephropathy
    D Post-streptococcal glomerulonephritis
    E Acute tubular necrosis

29. Which of the following is not a feature of Cushing's syndrome?

    A Central obesity
    B Poor wound healing
    C Hypotension
    D Striae
    E Proximal myopathy

30. A 24-year-old female is brought to A&E having fallen off a stage in a nightclub whilst under the influence of LSD. Her eyes open when the registrar squeezes her trapezius and she makes a few incomprehensible sounds. Her arms flex, wrists clench and legs extend and internally rotate in response to pain. What is her GCS?

    A 5
    B 7
    C 8
    D 9
    E 10

Answers

1. B

Hospital-acquired pneumonia (HAP) is defined as a pneumonia that develops more than 48 hrs after hospital admission. Causes of HAPs include Gram-negative enterobacteriaceae (e.g. *E. coli*), *S. aureus*, *Pseudomonas*, *Klebsiella*, *Bacterioides* and *Clostridia*. Causes of community-acquired pneumonia (CAP) include *S. pneumoniae* (most common), *H. influenzae*, *M. pneumoniae*, *Moraxella catarrhalis*, *Chlamydia* and *Legionella*.

2. D

A UTI is defined as the presence of a pure growth of >10^5 colony forming units per mL of fresh MSU. Therefore, an MSU should be sent for microscopy, culture and sensitivities (MC&S) to confirm a diagnosis of UTI. However, it is worth noting that up to 1 in 3 women with symptoms of UTI will have a negative MSU. If patients are symptomatic, a urine dipstick should be performed and, if nitrites or leukocytes are positive, empirical treatment should be commenced whilst awaiting the sensitivities from the MSU. U&Es are useful in assessing renal function in patients with upper urinary tract infections. Blood cultures may be performed if the patient is systemically unwell and showing features of urosepsis. CRP is an acute-phase protein that is elevated in most acute inflammatory or infectious conditions.

3. A

Gastroenteritis is a self-limiting disease that can be managed with bed rest and oral rehydration (to compensate for fluid and electrolyte losses from sweating, diarrhoea and vomiting). Hospital admission is required if the patient is vomiting and unable to retain oral fluids, has features of shock or is severely dehydrated (manifesting as confusion, weakness, tachycardia and hypotension). Antibiotics are only prescribed when the causative microorganism is identified by a stool culture. Anti-diarrhoeal agents are not usually necessary for the treatment of gastroenteritis, but they can be used for symptomatic relief in adults with mild-moderate disease.

4. B

Neurofibromatosis is an autosomal dominant condition resulting in the development of tumours in the nervous system. There are two main types. Type 1 mainly causes peripheral manifestations such as café-au-lait macules ('coffee-coloured, flat skin lesions'), axillary freckling, neurocutaneous fibromas, phaeochromocytomas and renal artery stenosis. Type 2 has mainly central features, such as bilateral vestibular schwannomas, meningiomas and gliomas.

Tuberous sclerosis is a genetic disease resulting in the formation of benign tumours in various organs across the body. The symptoms depend on the location of the tumours (e.g. brain — seizures; kidneys — haematuria). Xeroderma pigmentosum is a genetic disorder of DNA repair, which makes patients extremely susceptible to DNA damage by UV radiation and, leading to multiple skin cancers (e.g. melanoma, BCC). Dercum disease is characterised by the presence of several painful lipomas across the body.

5. C

The extra-articular features of ankylosing spondylitis can be remembered as the '5 As': **A**pical lung fibrosis, **A**myloidosis, **A**nterior uveitis, **A**chilles tendinitis and **A**ortic regurgitation.

Erythema ab igne is a reticulated rash caused by long-term exposure to heat. It is sometimes seen in chronic pancreatitis, hypothyroidism and lymphedema. Subcutaneous nodules are seen in rheumatoid arthritis. Tophi are deposits of monosodium urate crystals in joints, cartilage and bones. They occur in gout.

6. B

Haemopericardium is when blood accumulates in the pericardial sac leading to cardiac tamponade (compression of the heart). Haemopericardium can be caused by MI, trauma or aneurysm rupture. Cardiac tamponade is characterised by Beck's triad of signs: muffled heart sounds, raised JVP and hypotension (all of which are seen in this patient).

Acute heart failure tends to present with breathlessness and a cough productive of pink, frothy sputum. Pneumothorax, if severe, can result in a raised JVP and hypotension, however, the patient is also likely to be very breathless and examination will reveal a hyper-resonant area of the chest. Septic shock will cause hypotension, however, infectious symptoms (e.g. fever) are likely to be very prominent. Hypovolaemic shock will cause hypotension but JVP will be reduced and it is unlikely to cause muffled heart sounds.

7. D

Other than the chronic, dry cough, this patient has no symptoms or clinical signs of respiratory disease on examination. This makes asthma, interstitial lung disease, bronchiectasis and atypical pneumonia very unlikely. He has recently been diagnosed with hypertension, and, being under 55 years old, he is likely to have been prescribed an ACE inhibitor (e.g. ramipril) in accordance with the NICE guidelines. ACE inhibitors reduce the production of angiotensin II, leading to reduced sodium and water reabsorption in the kidneys and reduced vasoconstriction, which, ultimately, results in a reduction in blood pressure. ACE is also responsible for breaking down an inflammatory mediator called bradykinin. ACE inhibitors, therefore, lead to an accumulation of bradykinin in the lungs, which leads to a dry cough. Approximately, 10% of patients on ACE inhibitors will develop a chronic, dry cough.

8. D

Erythema nodusum is a panniculitis (inflammation of subcutaneous fat cells), which causes crops of red or violet dome-shaped nodules to appear on both shins (or occasionally on the thighs). They are tender and warm on palpation. Systemic symptoms (such as fever, malaise and arthralgia) may also be present. A helpful mnemonic to remember the causes of erythema nodusum is **LOST BUSH**:

— **L**eprosy, Lymphoma (non-hodgkins), Leukaemia
— **O**ral contraceptive (and pregnancy)
— **S**arcoidosis, Sulphonamides (and penicillins)

— TB, Toxoplasmosis
— Behçet's disease
— Ulcerative Colitis (and Crohn's disease)
— Salmonella (and Yersinia), Strep
— Histoplasmosis

9. A

This patient is experiencing acute-onset right upper quadrant pain and jaundice on a background of, what sounds like, biliary colic ('stabbing pain' after eating). Furthermore, the patient is Murphy's sign-positive, which is a classic feature of cholecystitis. Biliary colic occurs when a gallstone gets stuck in the common bile duct, resulting in contractions of the smooth muscle around the bile duct in an attempt to relieve the obstruction. Therefore, it suggests that this patient has gallstones. If a gallstone becomes infected, it can cause cholecystitis. The raised ALP and bilirubin indicates that the problem is within the biliary tract rather than being an intrinsic liver issue (such as viral hepatitis, which causes a rise in AST and ALT). Hepatocellular carcinoma is unlikely as this patient does not report any weight loss or any other systemic features of malignancy. Gilbert's syndrome is an autosomal recessive condition caused by reduced activity of the enzyme responsible for conjugating bilirubin. This results in episodes of asymptomatic jaundice, usually triggered by stress, exercise, lack of sleep, fasting and illness. LFTs tend to be normal in Gilbert's, except for a mildly elevated unconjugated bilirubin level.

10. A

Sickle cell disease is an autosomal recessive condition caused by a point mutation in the β-globin gene leading to the generation of abnormal haemoglobin — HbS. Hydrophobic interactions between HbS molecules leads to the formation of insoluble polymers, resulting in cell sickling. Sickle cells are less stable and more rigid and therefore are prone to destruction (with a lifespan of 20 days) and occluding small vessels. The patient is suffering from dactlylitis — painful inflammation of the digits due to a vaso-occlusive crisis. Other complications of sickle cell disease include autosplenectomy (infarction of the spleen leading to fibrosis and

204 SBAs in Medicine and Surgery

atrophy), sequestration crises (responsible for acute chest syndrome and priapism), haemolytic crisis (accelerated red cell breakdown) and aplastic crisis (triggered by parvovirus B19 infection). The inheritance patterns of some important diseases are listed in Question No. 1 and its respective answer from Paper 7.

11. C

This patient is in status epilepticus — a seizure lasting longer than 30 mins or repeated seizures without recovery or regain of consciousness in between. It is a medical emergency and should be treated as soon as a seizure lasts longer than 5 mins as there can be long-term consequences of waiting until 30 mins have passed (such as functional impairments due to neuronal injury and death). The patient's airway should be secured and high-flow oxygen should be administered. ECG, blood pressure and pulse oximetry monitors are attached, blood glucose is measured and IV access is established. A benzodiazepine is then administered in the form of IV lorazepam or PR diazepam (buccal midazolam is also used in the community setting). If the seizure persists, after 10 mins, they are started on a phenytoin infusion. Blood pressure and ECG are closely monitored because hypotension and arrhythmias are adverse effects of a rapid infusion of IV phenytoin. If the seizure still does not terminate after another 10 mins, IV thiopentone (general anaesthetic) can be used.

12. D

Confusion is a very common presenting complaint of hyponatraemia. It should be noted, however, that confusion is a very non-specific symptom, especially in the elderly (other causes include constipation, UTI and pneumonia). When considering causes of hyponatraemia, it is important to assess the patient's fluid status. Fluid status is not mentioned in this question, but the following causes should be kept in mind:

HYPERvolaemia: congestive cardiac failure, cirrhosis, nephrotic syndrome
EUvolaemia: adrenal insufficiency, SIADH, hypothyroidism
HYPOvolaemia: diarrhoea, vomiting, diuretics.

Aside from the confusion, the weight loss and haemoptysis in a heavy smoker should raise strong suspicion of lung cancer. Small cell lung cancer is the most common type of lung cancer in smokers, and it is associated with the ectopic production of two major hormones: ACTH and ADH. Ectopic ACTH would lead to Cushing's syndrome. Ectopic ADH (as is the case here), will lead to hyponatraemia.

Addison's disease would typically cause hyperkalaemia as well as hyponatraemia. In SBAs, buccal/palmar crease pigmentation and postural hypotension are commonly mentioned as presenting symptoms and signs of Addison's. There is nothing to suggest a diagnosis cirrhosis or congestive cardiac failure, furthermore there is no mention of fluid overload. Hypothyroid patients would have more hypothyroid symptoms (e.g. weight gain, depression, proximal myopathy) mentioned in the question.

13. B

The description of the chest pain as being 'sharp' suggests that this is pleuritic pain. The main causes of pleuritic chest pain can be remembered as the **5 Ps**: **P**E, **p**neumothorax, **p**neumonia, **p**ericarditis and **p**leurisy. The preceding flu-like illness makes this most likely to be pericarditis. The classic ECG feature of pericarditis is widespread ST elevation. This feature should not be mistaken with STEMI, because it would be impossible (or rather, extremely unlikely) to have an infarction affecting all regions of the heart at the same time.

ST elevation in II, III and aVF is a feature of inferior myocardial infarcts (caused by occlusion of the right coronary artery). ST depression is seen in NSTEMI. 'Tented T waves' is a buzzword used in many SBAs about ECG changes in hyperkalaemia. Absent P waves is found in several disturbances of rhythm, most notably atrial fibrillation and supraventricular tachycardia.

14. A

UTIs are much more common in women for two main anatomical reasons. Women have a shorter distance between their urethral opening and their bladder, meaning that there is a shorter distance for bacteria to travel to reach the bladder and establish an infection. Women also have a shorter distance between their urethral opening and their anus, which is a source of bacteria that can cause UTIs. Other risk factors include sexual activity, menopause, urinary tract abnormalities, immunosuppression and catheter use.

15. C

A chronic dry cough and shortness of breath in an individual of Afro-Caribbean origin, should get you thinking about sarcoidosis. Sarcoidosis is a disease of unknown cause in which non-caseating granulomas form in various parts of the body, most commonly the lungs. Erythema nodusum (tender violet nodules on the shin) is often seen in patients with sarcoidosis, although it is not specific to the condition. Bilateral hilar lymphadenopathy is the radiological hallmark of sarcoidosis, although it can also be caused by TB and lymphoma. Granulomatous tissue in sarcoidosis produces ectopic 1a-hydroxylase, which converts 25-hydroxy vitamin D3 to, the active, 1,25-dihydroxy vitamin D3 (calcitriol). This leads to excessive production of calcitriol which, in turn, leads to a rise in serum Ca^{2+}. Serum ACE levels will also be elevated in sarcoidosis, and is often measured to aid the diagnosis.

16. B

This patient's symptoms are consistent with inflammatory bowel disease (more likely to be Crohn's disease due to the absence of bloody diarrhoea), irritable bowel syndrome and coeliac disease. However, the rash on the patient's elbows is describing dermatitis herpetiformis, an extra-GI feature of coeliac disease. Serology for anti-tissue transglutaminase (anti-tTG) antibodies is the most useful diagnostic test for Coeliac disease as high titres of anti-tTG are found in almost all patients with the disease. Full blood count may show a microcytic anaemia.

Stool sample for MC&S would not be useful as this patient is presenting with a chronic history making gastroenteritis unlikely. As there are no signs of infection, a blood culture would be unnecessary. Barium follow-through is often used to visualise the extent of small-bowel involvement in Crohn's disease.

17. D

A breast cancer history can be difficult to take because there are several important risk factors that should be explored but are easy to forget. The main risk factors are age, a family history of breast or ovarian cancer, radiation to the chest and increased exposure to oestrogen (early menarche, late menopause, hormone replacement therapy, oral contraceptive pill). Pregnancy and breastfeeding reduce the risk of developing breast cancer by reducing the total number of menstrual cycles during a woman's lifetime.

18. B

An acutely painful and swollen joint on a background of systemic upset (e.g. fever, malaise) should be considered septic arthritis until proven otherwise. An urgent joint aspiration, for microscopy, culture and sensitivities, should be performed and treatment with empirical antibiotics should be commenced until sensitivities are known. Blood cultures may also be taken. The most common causative organisms are *S. aureus*, streptococci and *Neisseria gonorrhoeae* (this question lists *Neisseria meningitidis* as an option).

N. gonorrhoeae is a common cause of septic arthritis in young, sexually active adults. *H. influenzae* is a common cause in children. *E. coli* can cause septic arthritis in the elderly and IV drug users. TB is a rare cause of septic arthritis.

19. C

Tuning fork tests are not diagnostic; however, they do provide useful clues. There are two main tests: Weber's and Rinne's.

Rinne's Test – the prongs of a vibrating 512 Hz tuning fork are held in front of the patient's ear canal (testing air conduction), and then the base of the tuning fork is placed on the patient's mastoid process (testing bone conduction). The patient is then asked which is louder. Outcomes:

- Air Conduction > Bone Conduction (Rinne positive) = normal or sensorineural hearing loss
- Bone Conduction > Air Conduction (Rinne negative) = conductive hearing loss.

This is repeated in both ears.

Weber's Test — a vibrating 512 Hz tuning fork is placed on the patient's forehead and the patient is asked whether the sound is louder in either ear, or the same in both. Outcomes:

- Loudest in affected ear = conductive hearing loss
- Loudest in unaffected ear = sensorineural hearing loss
- Same in both ears = normal.

The patient in this question hears the sound loudest in her left ear during Weber's test — therefore, she has conductive hearing loss in the left ear or sensorineural hearing loss in the right ear. She is Rinne negative in both ears, thus eliminating conductive hearing loss as an option. This leaves sensorineural hearing loss in the right ear as the correct option.

20. A

Chronic kidney disease (CKD) is defined as >3 months of impaired renal function based on abnormal structure or function, or a GFR <60 mL/min/1.73m^2 for >3 months with or without evidence of kidney damage. Symptoms include anorexia, nausea and vomiting, pruritus, fatigue, peripheral oedema, muscle cramps and pulmonary oedema. These tend to occur once GFR <30.

21. B

Simplified outline of the management of acute heart failure:

1. Sit the patient upright (*not* lying them down)
2. Administer oxygen
3. Gain IV access and monitor ECG (treat arrhythmias)
4. IV Diamorphine
5. IV Furosemide
6. GTN spray or infusion
7. Consider CPAP if the patient's condition worsens.

Diamorphine, furosemide and GTN are venodilators which reduce venous return to the heart, thereby reducing preload, pulmonary venous congestion and pulmonary oedema. Diamorphine also serves as an anxiolytic.

22. A

Causes of the three main types of anaemia are as follows:

- **MICROcytic** — iron deficiency anaemia, anaemia of chronic disease, thalassemia, sideroblastic anaemia
- **NORMOcytic** — aplastic anaemia, haemolysis, post-haemorrhage, pregnancy, fluid overload
- **MACROcytic** — B12 deficiency, folate deficiency, drugs (e.g. methotrexate), alcohol excess, liver disease, myelodysplasia, hypothyroidism, multiple myeloma.

23. D

Superior vena cava syndrome (SVCS) is caused by compression of the superior vena cava, most commonly by lung tumours. Rarer causes include mediastinal lymphadenopathy and thymomas. The main features of SVCS are dyspnea, orthopnoea, swollen face and arms, plethora, cough and engorged neck and facial veins (raised and non-pulsatile JVP). SVCS can be identified using Pemberton's test — the patient is asked to lift their arms over their head for approximately 1 min, which leads to facial plethora, a raised non-pulsatile JVP and inspiratory stridor. This patient's 6-month history of haemoptysis and weight loss, in the context of SVCS, makes lung cancer very likely.

24. C

Acute glaucoma is caused by increased ocular pressure due to reduced outflow of aqueous humour. The obstruction to outflow can be due to the closing of the angle between the iris and the cornea. It most commonly affects the elderly, and presents with a painful red eye, vomiting, impaired vision and the perception of haloes around lights. Prompt diagnosis and treatment is essential, because acute glaucoma can lead to blindness.

Meningitis, migraine and subarachnoid haemorrhage are unlikely to cause such prominent eye signs. Cluster headaches can cause lacrimation and eye pain, however, it is unlikely to significantly impair vision. Furthermore, they tend to occur in 'clusters' — occurring every day at around the same time for a period of weeks/months. The clusters will be separated by pain-free periods.

25. A

In left ventricular systolic failure, the ejection fraction is low, which causes a reduced stroke volume and an increased end-diastolic volume. The high end-diastolic volume, following one weak contraction, stretches the ventricular muscle fibres which, by Starling's law, leads to a stronger subsequent contraction. This pattern of alternating strong and weak pulses is described as pulsus alternans.

Pulsus paradoxus refers to an abnormally large decrease in blood pressure and pulse amplitude during inspiration. Causes include constrictive peri-carditis and cardiac tamponade. A water-hammer pulse is a high-volume, collapsing pulse associated with aortic regurgitation. Pulsus parvus et tardus is a slow-rising pulse associated with aortic stenosis. Pulsus bisfe-riens refers to a biphasic pulse that has two peaks per cardiac cycle. It can be detected in HOCM and in patients with coexisting aortic regurgitation and aortic stenosis.

26. D

Obstructive sleep apnoea (OSA) is a disorder characterised by the inter-mittent collapse of the upper airways during sleep, resulting in episodes of apnoea ending with arousal. Most patients with OSA are overweight or obese — the extra weight around their airways makes it more likely that their airways will collapse. Patients with OSA will experience daytime sleepiness, however, they may not be aware that their sleep is disturbed because the arousal that terminates an apneic episode does not last long enough for the patient's brain to become aware of the arousal. So, despite being unaware of the arousal, the patient will remain in stage 1 and 2 (light) sleep without progressing to stage 3 and 4 (deep) sleep. Bed partners often complain of snoring. Patients are advised to lose weight and severe cases may be treated with CPAP (continuous positive airway pressure) via a nasal mask during sleep.

Narcolepsy is a rare condition in which patients experience intermittent sleep attacks. Cataplexy is characterised by sudden physical collapse with intact consciousness, stimulated by strong emotion or laughter. An absence seizure is a type of generalised seizure in which patients lose consciousness whilst postural muscle tone is maintained. It is more common in children. Central sleep apnoea occurs when the neural drive to breathe during sleep is impaired. It has many causes including stroke and heart failure.

27. C

The presence of HBsAb suggests that this patient has either been vaccinated or has cleared the virus after being infected. HBcAb IgG+ is only generated when infected and is not present in vaccinated individuals. Therefore, this patient has cleared a hepatitis B infection. Please refer to Question No. 5 and its respective answer from Paper 2 for a full explanation of hepatitis serology.

28. B

IgA nephropathy, also known as Berger's Disease, is the most common type of glomerulonephritis worldwide. It causes nephritic syndrome, which is characterised by a triad of proteinuria, haematuria and hypertension. The preceding pharyngitis is an important feature of this SBA. IgA nephropathy and post-streptococcal glomerulonephritis can both occur following a pharyngeal infection. A key difference is the interval between the infectious symptoms and the onset of glomerulonephritis. Post-streptococcal glomerulonephritis tends to occur 4–6 weeks after a streptococcal infection (e.g. streptococcal pharyngitis, cellulitis). Whereas IgA nephropathy tends to occur 5–7 days after the patient experiences symptoms of pharyngitis. Hypertension is more common in post-streptococcal glomerulonephritis, whereas heavy proteinuria and systemic symptoms, such as abdominal pain, skin rashes and arthritis, are more common in IgA nephropathy.

Minimal change disease (more common in children) and membranous nephropathy (more common in adults) are causes of nephrotic syndrome. Acute tubular necrosis (ATN) is the most common cause of intrinsic acute kidney injury (AKI). It typically results from renal hypoperfusion (e.g. due to congestive cardiac failure) or from the use of nephrotoxic drugs. ATN presents with reduced urine output and features of renal failure, such as fluid retention and nausea.

29. C

Aside from options A, B, D and E, other textbook features of Cushing's syndrome include moon face, thin skin, easy bruising and interscapular fat pad (often referred to as a 'buffalo hump'). Cushing's syndrome causes hypertension. The 11b-hydroxysteroid dehydrogenase enzyme in the kidneys, which converts cortisol into, the inactive, cortisone, normally prevents cortisol from having a mineralocorticoid effect. However, in Cushing's syndrome, the high cortisol levels overwhelm this protective system, meaning that cortisol exerts a mineralocorticoid effect — increasing salt and water reabsorption, thereby increasing blood pressure.

30. B

The Glasgow Coma Scale (GCS) is used to record the level of consciousness of a patient following head trauma. GCS measures three functions: eye opening, verbal response and motor response. The total of these three components fall between 3 (completely unresponsive) and 15, with a score of 8 or less being considered as comatose. Refer to Question No. 3 and its respective answer from Paper 1 for the breakdown of GCS. This patient's eyes opened in response to pain (2), she made incomprehensible sounds (2) and her motor response was decorticate (3) — giving a total of 7.

Paper 9

Questions

1. An 8-year-old girl visits her GP, with her mother, 4 weeks after being prescribed antibiotics for a sore throat. Her urine has become tea-coloured and she has been feeling nauseous with a headache. Urinalysis reveals proteinuria and haematuria and her blood pressure is 137/72 mm Hg. A diagnosis of post-infectious glomerulonephritis is suspected. Which organism is most likely responsible?

   A *Streptococcus agalactiae*
   B *Streptococcus pyogenes*
   C *Escherichia coli*
   D *Diphtheria*
   E *Bordetella pertussis*

2. Which of the following drugs is not used in the long-term management of chronic heart failure?

   A Indomethacin
   B Carvedilol
   C Spironolactone
   D Candesartan
   E Digoxin

3. A 32-year-old man has been suffering from worsening shortness of breath over the past 5 months. He used to be very physically active, but, recently, he has become breathless whilst doing relatively low intensity tasks such as walking to the bus stop. He has also developed a chronic cough, productive of clear sputum. He regularly visits the hospital to monitor his liver function because of a 'liver disease' that he has had since he was a child. He has never smoked and does not drink alcohol. What is the most likely diagnosis?

    A COPD
    B Autoimmune hepatitis
    C α_1 antitrypsin deficiency
    D Haemochromatosis
    E Wilson's disease

4. A 55-year-old woman presents with a 2-month history of jaundice and right upper quadrant pain. She has a history of ulcerative colitis. LFTs and serology are requested:

ALP: 390 iU/L (30–150)
AST: 40 iU/L (5–35)
ALT: 40 iU/L (5–35)
GGT: 150 iU/L (7–32)
pANCA: Positive

What is the most likely diagnosis?

    A Haemochromatosis
    B Primary biliary cirrhosis
    C Primary sclerosing cholangitis
    D Autoimmune hepatitis
    E Wilson's disease

5. An 89-year-old woman is brought into A&E after she suddenly became very disorientated and was unable to recognise her own son.

On examination, she is blind in the left half of her visual field. An ischaemic stroke is suspected. Which artery is most likely to be involved?

    A Right anterior cerebral artery
    B Right posterior cerebral artery
    C Left posterior cerebral artery
    D Right middle cerebral artery
    E Left middle cerebral artery

6. Which of the following conditions is strongly associated with Giant Cell Arteritis?

    A Takayasu's aortitis
    B Myalgic encephalomyelitis
    C Fibromyalgia
    D Polymyalgia rheumatic
    E Polymyositis

7. A 58-year-old woman presents with a scaly rash around her right nipple. She says that the rash has been there for the last 3 weeks. On examination, there is a crusty rash around her right nipple and palpation reveals a firm lump just below the areola that appears to be tethered to surrounding tissues. What is the most likely diagnosis?

    A Intraductal papilloma
    B Phyllodes tumour
    C Paget's disease of the breast
    D Breast abscess
    E Fibroadenoma

8. A 43-year-old businesswoman has had a TIA. Soon after landing in the UK from a business trip to Australia, she suddenly became unable to move her right arm. She began slurring her speech, the right side of her face started drooping and she temporarily lost vision in her right

eye. She adds that she experienced some pain in her right leg as she was disembarking the plane, however, she assumed it was a muscle strain from wearing high-heels for several days. What underlying defect is most likely to have caused her TIA?

    A Atrial fibrillation
    B Atrial septal defect
    C Carotid atherosclerosis
    D Infective endocarditis
    E Prosthetic heart valve

9. Which of the following is not a recognised cause of acute pancreatitis?

    A Hyperlipidaemia
    B Hypothermia
    C Hypocalcaemia
    D Mumps
    E Azathioprine

10. A 34-year-old man is brought to A&E having collapsed in a shopping mall. He did not lose consciousness but mentioned that he felt dizzy and could feel his 'heart racing'. He has a past medical history of asthma. His ECG shows a regular narrow complex tachycardia with no visible P waves. Vagal manoeuvres failed to terminate the tachycardia. What is the next most appropriate step in the management of this patient?

    A Verapamil
    B Amiodarone
    C Adenosine
    D Bisoprolol
    E Flecainide

11. Which of the following is a cause of primary amenorrhoea?

    A Prolactinoma
    B Pregnancy

C Haemochromatosis

D Polycystic ovarian syndrome

E Turner syndrome

12. In which part of the nephron does bendroflumethiazide have its effect?

A Proximal convoluted tubule

B Descending limb of the loop of Henle

C Ascending limb of the loop of Henle

D Distal convoluted tubule

E Collecting duct

13. A 62-year-old heavy smoker is being investigated for lung cancer having presented with a 4-month history of unintentional weight loss, haemoptysis and fatigue. He claims that his voice has become hoarse and a junior doctor adds that he has a textbook 'bovine cough'. In which part of the lung is the tumour most likely to be found?

A Left apex

B Right middle lobe

C Right base

D Left base

E Pleura

14. Which of the following most accurately describes the sodium and potassium requirements of a 70 kg man over a 24-hr period?

A 100 mmol Na^+ and 40–50 mmol K^+

B 120 mmol Na^+ and 5–10 mmol K^+

C 120 mmol Na^+ and 10–20 mmol K^+

D 120 mmol Na^+ and 60–70 mmol K^+

E 140 mmol Na^+ and 60–70 mmol K^+

15. A 27-year-old female presents to her GP complaining of an episode of painful loss of vision that lasted 1 day and resolved spontaneously. Six months ago, she lost sensation across the lateral half of her left leg

which also resolved spontaneously. Which of the following would
you expect to see in her diagnostic work up?

    A Bence Jones proteins
    B Oligoclonal bands on CSF electrophoresis
    C High CSF protein
    D Xanthochromia
    E Raised ICP

16. Which of the following is an acquired cause of long QT syndrome?

    A Romano–Ward syndrome
    B Hyponatraemia
    C Hyperkalaemia
    D Hypomagnesaemia
    E Hypercalcaemia

17. A 70-year-old man presents with a 3-month history of polyuria.
He has been urinating up to 12 times per day and has also experienced
some constipation, abdominal pain and back pain. More recently, he
has noticed that his face appears 'puffier' than usual and his ankles are
swollen. He is on citalopram to treat his depression and takes no other
regular medications. Blood tests reveal: ESR = 64 mm/hr (<22).
Urinalysis reveals:

Protein: Positive
Blood: Negative 24-hr urine protein (g): 9.8 (<3.5)

What is the most likely diagnosis?

    A Cushing's syndrome
    B Amyloidosis
    C Glomerulonephritis
    D Malignancy
    E Congestive cardiac failure

18. What is the most common cause of urinary tract infections?

    A *Staphylococcus aureus*
    B *Staphylococcus saprophyticus*
    C *Enterococcus faecalis*
    D *Escherichia coli*
    E *Klebsiella pneumonia*

19. A 36-year-old man presents to his GP with a 1-month history of short-ness of breath on exertion. He has also experienced a low-grade fever and a dry cough. He has a past medical history of HIV. A pulse oxi-meter is attached showing an oxygen saturation of 97% at rest. The patient is then asked to walk up and down the room a few times and his oxygen saturation drops to 88%. What is the most likely diagnosis?

    A Interstitial lung disease
    B Pulmonary embolism
    C *Pneumocystis jirovecii* pneumonia
    D Mycobacterium avium complex
    E Bronchiectasis

20. An 88-year-old care home resident is receiving oral clarithromycin to treat a chest infection. She develops profuse watery diarrhoea and her temperature rises to 38.2°C. She has vomited three times and is expe-riencing diffuse abdominal discomfort. A stool sample is positive for *Clostridium difficile* toxin. Which antibiotic should be given to this patient?

    A Co-amoxiclav
    B Penicillin
    C Metronidazole
    D Ciprofloxacin
    E Tetracycline

21. What is another name for target cells?

    A Codocyte
    B Dacrocyte
    C Spherocyte
    D Reticulocyte
    E Schistocyte

22. A 34-year-old man with Marfan's syndrome, comes to A&E having experienced a sudden tearing chest pain. He adds that the pain seems to move to his back. On examination, an early diastolic murmur is heard over the aortic valve and unequal arm pulses are palpated. What is the most likely diagnosis?

    A Ruptured aortic aneurysm
    B Coarctation of the aorta
    C Aortic dissection
    D Myocardial infarction
    E Tension pneumothorax

23. Which set of spirometry results is most likely to be seen in a patient with COPD?

    A FEV1 > 0.8 and FEV1:FVC > 0.7
    B FEV1 < 0.8 and FEV1:FVC < 0.7
    C FEV1 > 0.8 and FEV1:FVC < 0.7
    D FEV1 < 0.8 and FEV1:FVC > 0.7
    E Impossible to tell without FVC measurement

24. A 15-year-old boy arrives at A&E with sudden-onset pain and swelling in his scrotum, which began 2 hrs ago whilst playing a rugby match. He also starts vomiting and complains of pain in his right iliac fossa. On examination, his right hemiscrotum is red and swollen. What is the most appropriate first step in his management?

    A Doppler ultrasound of the testes
    B CT scan

C Exploratory surgery
D Empirical antibiotics
E Abdominal X-ray

25. Which scoring system is used to determine a patient's risk of developing pressure sores?

   A GRACE score
   B ABCD^2 score
   C Ranson score
   D Waterlow score
   E Rockall score

26. A 36-year-old man presents with a 3-week history of fatigue, frequent urination and excessive thirst. He also mentions that he has been unable to take part in his weekly 5-a-side football sessions for the past month because his 'muscles feel weak'. The patient's notes reveal that, during a previous appointment 6 months ago, his blood pressure was measured at 164/98 mm Hg. He was offered a follow-up appointment to discuss management options, however, he did not attend. The GP measures the patient's blood pressure again, and it is 172/102 mm Hg. What would you expect to see on the ECG of this patient?

   A Tented T waves
   B Absent P waves
   C ST elevation
   D J waves
   E U waves

27. A 40-year-old man is brought into A&E after he was found lying unconscious on the side of the road with an empty bottle of whisky next to him. Once he regains consciousness, he starts yelling at the ward staff expressing that he thinks he has been kidnapped and is being held hostage. He jumps out of bed, but finds it difficult to walk. He has a wide-based gait and he is taking small steps. Given

the most likely diagnosis, what should form part of the immediate management?

  A Acamprosate
  B Chlordiazepoxide
  C Thiamine
  D Naloxone
  E Disulfiram

28. Which of the following is not a reversible cause of cardiac arrest?

  A Hypothermia
  B Tension pneumothorax
  C Cardiac tamponade
  D Hypokalaemia
  E Pleurisy

29. A 44-year-old woman presents with right upper quadrant pain that radiates to the tip of her right shoulder with an intermittent fever, severe chills and sweats. She has also recently experienced hiccups, breathlessness and a dry cough. On examination, there is tenderness over the 8th to 11th ribs on the right side and dullness to percussion, diminished breath sounds and reduced chest expansion over the lower zone of the right lung. Ten days prior to the onset of symptoms, she had a laparoscopic appendectomy. What is the most likely diagnosis?

  A Acute cholangitis
  B Basal pneumonia
  C Subphrenic abscess
  D Atelectasis
  E Liver abscess

30. Which of the following endocrine conditions can cause hyperprolactinaemia?

    A Cushing's syndrome
    B Phaeochromocytoma
    C Addison's disease
    D Graves' disease
    E Hypothyroidism

Answers

1. B

Post-infectious glomerulonephritis is most common in children and occurs 1–12 weeks after a streptococcal infection of the pharynx (strep throat) or skin. Strep throat is caused by *Streptococcus pyogenes* (group A streptococcus), transmitted via the oral secretions of an infected individual. Deposition of immune complexes in the glomeruli leads to nephritic syndrome, characterised by haematuria (which may be macroscopic, hence the tea-coloured urine), proteinuria, hypertension and oliguria. Systemic symptoms such as fever, nausea and headache may also be present.

2. A

NSAIDs, such as indomethacin, are contraindicated in chronic heart failure because they can cause sodium and water retention, peripheral vasoconstriction and worsening heart failure. Furthermore, NSAIDs are nephrotoxic which could further decrease the function of hypoperfused kidneys in chronic heart failure.

The management of chronic heart failure primarily involves five drugs/drug classes: diuretics, ACE inhibitors, beta-blockers, spironolactone and digoxin. Diuretics can reduce sodium and fluid absorption, leading to symptomatic relief and a reduced mortality. ACE inhibitors prevent adverse cardiac remodelling, and have a positive effect on survival. Angiotensin receptor blockers (ARBs e.g. candesartan) can be used if ACE inhibitors are not tolerated. Beta-blockers (e.g. carvedilol) are used with caution because maintaining the sympathetic drive to the heart is vital for preserving cardiac function, however, they have been shown to improve survival. Spironolactone is a potassium-sparing diuretic, which can further improve survival. Digoxin provides symptomatic relief, however, it does not improve survival. Vasodilators such as hydralazine and isosorbide dinitrite are sometimes used in Afro-Caribbean patients with heart failure.

3. C

α_1 antitrypsin (A1AT) is a serine protease inhibitor produced by the liver, which is responsible for protecting body tissues from the harmful action of neutrophil elastase, a protease produced by neutrophils. A1AT deficiency is an inherited condition characterised by the production of much lower levels of A1AT by the liver. This means that the lungs are vulnerable to damage by neutrophil elastase — over time, this leads to emphysema. In patients with A1AT deficiency, the secretion of A1AT by liver cells is defective, leading to an accumulation of A1AT in the liver, ultimately resulting in cirrhosis. The degree to which patients with A1AT deficiency are affected varies, but it typically presents with cirrhosis and emphysema at a young age.

4. C

Gradual onset jaundice and right upper quadrant pain, along with an elevated ALP and GGT, mild transaminitis and positive pANCA is strongly suggestive of primary sclerosing cholangitis (PSC). This is further supported by the patient's history of ulcerative colitis, which is closely linked with PSC.

Primary biliary cirrhosis (PBC) is associated with anti-mitochondrial antibodies (AMA) and tends to be asymptomatic with a persistently elevated ALP. Haemochromatosis is a disease of iron metabolism presenting with a triad of bronzed skin, hepatomegaly and diabetes mellitus. Although autoimmune hepatitis also presents insidiously with jaundice and right upper quadrant pain, you would expect AST and ALT to be much higher than it is in this patient. Furthermore, serology in autoimmune hepatitis is likely to detect anti-nuclear antibodies (ANA), anti-smooth muscle antibodies (ASMA), anti-liver soluble antigen antibodies (ASLA — type 1 autoimmune hepatitis) or antibodies against liver/kidney microsome type 1 (anti-LKM1 — type 2 autoimmune hepatitis). Wilson's disease is a disorder of copper metabolism, presenting with hepatic, neurological, psychiatric and ocular findings.

5. B

The inability to recognise faces is known as prosopagnosia, which can result from damage to the occipital lobes due to an occlusion in the posterior cerebral artery (PCA). Homonymous hemianopia is also a feature of occlusion of the PCA. For more information on stroke territories, refer to Question No. 24 and its respective answer from Paper 2.

6. D

Giant cell arteritis (GCA), also known as temporal arteritis, is a large-vessel vasculitis of unknown cause. It presents with a headache, temporal artery and scalp tenderness, jaw claudication and it can cause sudden blindness (usually in one eye). 50% of GCA patients also have polymyalgia rheumatica (PMR) — an inflammatory disease of unknown cause, which presents with bilateral tenderness, aching and stiffness in the shoulder and pelvic girdle area. Empirical treatment with high-dose oral prednisolone should be commenced if there is any suspicion of GCA, and ESR can be used as a screening tool. Temporal artery biopsy is the gold standard for diagnosis of GCA, however, the biopsy sample may not be taken from an area of inflammation so it may not always be conclusive.

7. C

Paget's disease of the breast is an eczema-like hardening of the skin overlying the nipple. It usually occurs secondary to an underlying breast cancer. This should not be confused with Paget's disease of the bone.

An intraductal papilloma is a benign tumour that forms within the milk ducts of the breast. It presents as a small breast lump near the nipple, often accompanied by a blood-stained nipple discharge. A Phyllodes tumour is a rare fibroepithelial breast tumour that grows rapidly and usually presents as a breast lump. Breast abscesses can be divided into lactational (occurring in women who are breastfeeding) and non-lactational (typically occurring in 30–60-year-old women who smoke). It presents with a painful breast swelling which may have an overlying area of erythema. These patients are also likely to have a fever and feel generally unwell. A fibroadenoma is a benign tumour of the collagenous tissue within the breast lobule that typically occurs in younger women. The lumps are usually firm, smooth, mobile and painless.

8. B

TIAs are most frequently caused by emboli from atrial fibrillation or carotid atherosclerosis. Other sources of emboli include valve vegetations in infective endocarditis and prosthetic heart valves. This patient describes pain in her right leg soon after disembarking a long-haul flight — likely to be a DVT. In a small minority of patients, instead of causing a PE, a DVT can cause a TIA or stroke by passing through a septal defect in the heart, thereby, bypassing the lungs and travelling to the brain. This phenomenon is known as a paradoxical embolism.

9. C

The causes of acute pancreatitis can be remembered using the mnemonic **GET SMASHED**: **G**allstones, **E**thanol, **T**rauma, **S**teroids, **M**umps, **A**utoimmune, **S**corpion venom, **H**yperlipidaemia/Hypothermia/ Hypercalcaemia, **E**RCP and **D**rugs (e.g. azathioprine, sodium valproate). Gallstones and alcohol are responsible for around 80% of cases. N.B. Hypercalcaemia can cause acute pancreatitis, but acute pancreatitis can lead to hypocalcaemia due to the binding of digested lipids to calcium (a process called saponification).

10. A

Following the diagnosis of SVT based on ECG findings, the stepwise management of a stable patient with SVT begins by attempting vagal manoeuvres (e.g. Valsalva manoeuvre). If the vagal manoeuvres fail, a 6 mg IV bolus of adenosine should be administered. If the first attempt fails, repeat the 6 mg bolus. If this fails, administer a 12 mg IV bolus. Amiodarone may be used if adenosine is ineffective. Adenosine is contraindicated in asthmatics as it can precipitate bronchospasm. In this case, 2.5–5 mg of verapamil is used instead.

Bisoprolol is a beta-blocker that is often used for rate control in patients with AF. Flecainide is an anti-arrhythmic used for rhythm control in AF.

11. E

Amenorrhoea can be described as primary (menstruation has never occurred) or secondary (menstruation has stopped for at least 6 months in

a patient who has previously menstruated). Turner syndrome, a chromosomal abnormality with the genotype 45 X, leads to primary amenorrhoea.
Prolactinoma, pregnancy, haemochromatosis and polycystic ovarian syndrome can cease menstruation in women have menstruated before — thus
causing secondary amenorrhoea.

12. D

Bendroflumethiazide is a thiazide diuretic which inhibits the Na^+/Cl^-
transporter in the distal convoluted tubule leading to increased sodium and
water excretion. Loop diuretics (e.g. furosemide) inhibit the $Na^+/K^+/Cl^-$
triple transporter in the thick ascending limb of the loop of Henle.
Potassium-sparing diuretics (e.g. spironolactone) are aldosterone antagonists which inhibit aldosterone-mediated sodium reabsorption in the
collecting ducts. Amiloride blocks sodium channels within the collecting
tubules and has a similar effect to spironolactone. Osmotic diuretics are
solutes that are freely filtered but poorly reabsorbed, so they remain in the
filtrate and exert an osmotic pressure that holds water within the tubules,
thereby reducing water reabsorption. Carbonic anhydrase inhibitors act on
the proximal convoluted tubule to increase bicarbonate excretion, which,
in turn, increases sodium excretion.

13. A

The recurrent laryngeal nerves innervate all the intrinsic muscles of the
larynx, except the cricothyroid muscles, and are responsible for control-
ling the voice. The recurrent laryngeal nerves branch off the vagus nerve
in the thorax, and then run superiorly towards the laryngeal muscles (ety-
mology: re- = back; currere = to run). Recurrent laryngeal nerve injury can
result in a hoarse voice and a 'bovine' cough. Apical lung tumours can
compress the recurrent laryngeal nerve (usually on the left side because
the left recurrent laryngeal nerve branches off the vagus nerve more infe-
riorly) and cause these symptoms. Neck surgery (e.g. thyroidectomy) is
another common cause of recurrent laryngeal nerve injury.

14. E

The fluid and electrolyte demands of the human body are dependent on
many factors, including weight. A 70 kg man is used as a reference in the

calculation of many normal ranges. These reference values are important in patients who are nil-by-mouth and require parenteral administration of fluids and electrolytes. A 70 kg man has a daily sodium and potassium requirement of 140 mmol and 60–70 mmol, respectively.

15. B

This young patient has experienced two episodes of neurological symptoms that are distanced in time (occurred on two different occasions) and space (two different parts of the central nervous system affected, in this case, the optic nerve and a sensory nerve). This is highly suggestive of multiple sclerosis (MS). The diagnosis of MS is heavily based on the clinical history and there is no straight-forward diagnostic test. However, CSF electrophoresis may show oligoclonal bands and an MRI scan may show sclerotic plaques that may or may not correspond with the neurological symptoms experienced by the patient.

Bence-Jones proteins are immunoglobulin light chains which are found in the urine of patients with multiple myeloma. High CSF protein is a feature of Guillain–Barré syndrome. Xanthochromia is a 'straw-coloured' discoloration of the CSF seen when performing a lumbar puncture. It is caused by the breakdown of red blood cells in the CSF and it is most commonly referred to in the context of subarachnoid haemorrhage. Xanthochromia will be present from 12 hrs to 12 days after onset of a subarachnoid haemorrhage. Raised ICP can be caused by several different conditions but it is not commonly associated with MS.

16. D

Long QT syndrome is a dangerous heart condition that increases the risk of potentially fatal arrhythmias such as torsades de pointes and ventricular fibrillation. The main acquired causes of long QT syndrome are hypokalaemia and hypomagnesaemia. Inherited causes include Romano–Ward syndrome and Jervell and Lange-Nielsen syndrome.

17. B

This is quite a difficult question and requires a stepwise approach. Firstly, the urinalysis results show no blood and high protein in the patient's urine.

This is suggestive of nephrotic syndrome — characterised by a triad of proteinuria (>3.5 g/day), hypoalbuminaemia and oedema ('puffier' face and swollen ankles). There are many causes of nephrotic syndrome so it, in itself, is not a diagnosis. The patient has experienced polyuria, constipation, abdominal pain, back pain and depression, which is in keeping with the famous '*stones, bones, abdominal groans, thrones and psychiatric overtones*' mnemonic for hypercalcaemia. Hypercalcaemia with back pain and a raised ESR is suggestive of multiple myeloma — a condition characterised by proliferation of plasma cells resulting in bone lesions and the production of a monoclonal immunoglobulin (Ig). It has four main features, which can be remembered using the mnemonic '**CRAB**': Calcium (hypercalcaemia), Renal failure, Anaemia, Bone pain. Amyloidosis is a condition caused by the deposition of abnormal proteins (amyloid fibrils) in tissues, leading to tissue dysfunction. Ig light chains are a precursor for amyloid fibrils, so multiple myeloma can lead to amyloidosis. The deposition of amyloid fibrils in the kidneys leads to nephrotic syndrome.

This patient has some features which could suggest a diagnosis of malignancy (bone pain and hypercalcaemia), congestive cardiac failure (ankle swelling), glomerulonephritis (proteinuria — however, the absence of haematuria makes this less likely) and Cushing's syndrome (puffy face and depression). Nonetheless, the rest of the clinical picture does not match any of these diagnoses so make sure you do not anchor yourself onto buzzwords (e.g. 'puffier' face) and ignore the rest of the information provided in the SBA. Carefully consider every detail provided about the patient and how that impacts your answer.

18. D

A UTI is defined as the presence of a pure growth of $>10^5$ colony forming units per mL of fresh MSU. However, it is worth noting that up to 1 in 3 women with symptoms of UTI will have a negative MSU. It is a very common condition that mainly affects women. Although the term 'UTI' colloquially refers to cystitis, it is a broad term that also encompasses pyelonephritis (a more serious infection of the upper urinary tract). Cystitis usually presents with frequency, dysuria, urgency and suprapubic pain.

Pyelonephritis causes high fevers, rigors, vomiting and loin pain. It can lead to AKI and sepsis. *E. coli* is the most common cause of UTI. Other causative organisms include *P. mirabilis*, *K. pneumoniae* and *S. saprophyticus*.

19. C

Pneumocystis jirovecii is a fungus that causes pneumonia in immunocompromised patients (e.g. HIV-positive patients). It presents with a dry cough, exertional dyspnoea and fever. On examination, the patient is often asked to walk up and down the room, whilst attached to a pulse oximeter, to demonstrate oxygen desaturation on exertion. A chest X-ray may be normal, or it may show bilateral pulmonary infiltrates. Diagnosis is confirmed by visualising the organism in a sputum, bronchoalveolar lavage or lung biopsy specimen. It is treated with high-dose co-trimoxazole and preventative measures are taken in HIV-positive patients when their CD4 count drops below 200×10^6/L.

Interstitial lung disease causes similar symptoms to *Pneumocystis* pneumonia but it doesn't cause such dramatic desaturation on exertion and it is not strongly associated with HIV. Bronchiectasis causes chronic shortness of breath but is usually accompanied by a cough productive of large volumes of purulent sputum. Mycobacterium avium complex (MAC) is a disease that affects HIV patients with very low CD4 counts. It has a similar presentation to TB. PE causes acute-onset shortness of breath.

20. C

C. difficile is present amongst the commensal colonic flora of 1/30 adults. Its harmful effects are mitigated by the presence of millions of competing commensal bacteria. Antibiotic use can eliminate these competing bacteria leading to an overgrowth of *C. difficile*. The release of toxins by *C. difficile* leads to extensive inflammation and disruption of the brush border membrane of the colon, resulting in what is known as pseudomembranous colitis. This usually presents with explosive diarrhoea. *C. difficile* is spread via the faecal-oral route and forms spores that can persist on unclean surfaces covered with small amounts of faecal matter. Poor hygiene practice by healthcare workers is a major mode of transmission of *C. difficile* between patients. It is treated with oral metronidazole or vancomycin.

21. A

Codocyte = Target cell (associated with liver disease and hyposplenism)

Dacrocyte = Tear-drop cell (associated with myelofibrosis)

Spherocyte = a small, spherical red blood cell (associated with hereditary spherocytosis and autoimmune haemolytic anaemia)

Reticulocyte = an immature red blood cell showing a basophilic reticulum when stained (a high reticulocyte count indicates increased red blood cell production activity in response to, for example, blood loss or haemolytic anaemia)

Schistocyte = red cell fragment (sign of intravascular haemolysis e.g. due to artificial heart valves or MAHA).

22. C

An aortic dissection occurs when blood tears the inner layer of the aorta, the tunica intima, and enters the tunica media, leading to a split between the inner and outer tunica media. This forms a 'false lumen' that can extend along the aorta and its branches. Aortic dissection usually presents with sudden, tearing chest pain that radiates to the back (usually between the shoulder blades). If the tear spreads along the branches of the aorta, it can lead to serious complications, depending on the arteries involved, such as strokes (carotid artery), MI (coronary arteries) and renal failure (renal artery). Risk factors include hypertension, atherosclerosis and connective tissue disease (e.g. Marfan's syndrome). There are two main types of aortic dissection according to the Stanford Classification: Type A = involves the ascending aorta; Type B = no involvement of the ascending aorta. A dissection that spreads towards the heart can cause aortic regurgitation (giving rise to the early diastolic murmur heard in this patient). A dissection proximal to the left subclavian artery will cause unequal arm pulses.

Coarctation of the aorta is a congenital narrowing of the aorta — a cause of secondary hypertension. Ruptured aortic aneurysms usually present with acute abdominal pain and circulatory collapse.

23. B

COPD is an obstructive respiratory disease resulting in an increase in airway resistance. The FEV1 is the volume exhaled during the first second of a forced expiratory manoeuvre — it is reduced in COPD because the narrowed airways create increased resistance to airflow. Forced vital capacity (FVC) is the total volume of air exhaled during a forced expiratory manoeuvre. A decrease in FEV1 results in a consequent drop in the FEV1:FVC ratio. According to NICE, COPD can be diagnosed when spirometry results show FEV1 < 0.8 and FEV1:FVC < 0.7.

FEV1 < 0.8 and FEV1:FVC > 0.7 is the typical pattern seen in restrictive lung disease, in which both FEV1 and FVC are reduced, however, the decrease in FVC is greater than that of FEV1, resulting in a normal or raised FEV1:FVC ratio.

24. C

Testicular torsion is a surgical emergency in which the spermatic cord twists resulting in venous outflow obstruction which progresses to arterial occlusion and testicular infarction. It typically presents with acute scrotal pain, abdominal pain and nausea and vomiting. The main risk factor for testicular torsion is a congenital abnormality known as the 'bell-clapper' deformity. Patients with suspected testicular torsion should be referred immediately for exploratory surgery. Exploration within 6 hrs of onset is necessary to maximise the chances of saving the testicle. Doppler ultrasound may show reduced blood flow to the testicle, however, this should not delay surgery. During the operation, the testicle will be twisted back into position and both testicles will be tethered to the scrotum to prevent recurrence. The cremasteric reflex is a useful test when examining a patient with testicular torsion. It is elicited by lightly stroking the inner thigh, which normally causes ipsilateral contraction of the cremaster muscle that pulls up the testis. The cremasteric reflex is absent in testicular torsion. Although it is not a particularly specific test, the presence of the cremasteric reflex makes testicular torsion very unlikely.

Epididymitis, inflammation of the epididymis caused by infection, is an important differential for acute scrotal pain. However, it is less acute than testicular torsion and will feature other signs of infection such as penile discharge and fever.

25. D

Pressure sores are extremely common in hospitalised or bed-bound patients. They occur due to constant pressure limiting blood flow to the skin, resulting in tissue damage. The risk of developing pressure sores is assessed using the Waterlow score.

The GRACE score allows triaging of patients with NSTEMI and unstable angina. The ABCD^2 score assesses the risk of having a stroke in patients who have had a TIA. The Ranson score is used to grade the severity of pancreatitis. However, the Glasgow score is more commonly used in the UK. The Rockall score is used to predict risk of re-bleed and mortality in patients that have suffered an upper GI bleed.

26. E

This patient has Conn's syndrome — a condition in which an aldosterone-secreting adenoma leads to inappropriately elevated aldosterone levels. The excessive sodium reabsorption and potassium excretion caused by the high aldosterone leads to hypertension and hypokalaemia. Hypokalaemia induces nephrogenic diabetes insipidus, which, consequently, leads to polyuria and polydipsia. Furthermore, muscle weakness is another feature of hypokalaemia. The main ECG features of hypokalaemia are U waves, ST depression, flattened T waves and prolonged PR interval. In any young patient presenting with hypertension, consider secondary causes such as Conn's syndrome, coarctation of the aorta and renal artery stenosis.

Tented T waves are a feature of hyperkalaemia. Absent P waves can be seen in several different conditions, most notably atrial fibrillation and supraventricular tachycardia. J waves (sometimes referred to as Osborn waves) are seen in hypothermia.

27. C

This patient has Wernicke's encephalopathy, a disease caused by biochemical damage to the central nervous system. It results from thiamine deficiency which typically occurs in alcoholics and the chronically malnourished. It is characterised by a triad of ophthalmoplegia, ataxia (wide-based gait with cerebellar signs) and confusion. Other features include memory loss, hallucinations, abnormal reflexes, weakness, hypothermia and hypotension. It is a medical emergency that requires treatment with IV thiamine to avoid progression to Korsakoff's psychosis, which is irreversible. 85% of patients, if left untreated, will develop Korsakoff's psychosis.

Acamprosate and disulfiram are used to treat alcohol dependence. Chlordiazepoxide is used to treat alcohol withdrawal. Naloxone is an antidote for opioid overdose.

28. E

The reversible causes of cardiac arrest can be remembered as 'the 4Hs and 4Ts':

Hypoxia
Hypothermia
Hypovolaemia
Hypokalaemia/Hyperkalaemia
Toxic
Thromboembolic
Tension pneumothorax
Tamponade

29. C

Upper abdominal pain radiating to the shoulder tip with a swinging fever in the days/weeks following abdominal surgery is suggestive of a subphrenic abscess. These are localised collections of pus, commonly underneath the right or left hemidiaphragm, which usually occur following a breach in the integrity of the peritoneum (e.g. perforated viscus, bowel surgery). Patients may also complain of malaise, weight loss, nausea, hiccups (due to diaphragmatic irritation by the abscess), a dry cough and shoulder tip pain (referred pain) on the affected side. The patient's respiratory symptoms are likely to be due to a pleural effusion. Abdominal CT or ultrasound are the preferred imaging modalities for visualising an abscess. FBC can aid diagnosis by showing leukocytosis and a chest X-ray will reveal a raised hemidiaphragm and a pleural effusion.

Liver abscesses can present similarly, but gastrointestinal signs such as hepatomegaly and jaundice will be more prominent, and respiratory symptoms are unlikely. Acute cholangitis is characterised by Charcot's triad: right upper quadrant pain, jaundice and fever with rigors. Although basal pneumonia may present with similar respiratory signs and right upper quadrant pain, it is also likely to cause a productive cough and pleuritic chest pain.

Atelectasis (partial lung collapse) can occur as a complication of a subphrenic abscess, however, it does not correspond with the clinical scenario described.

30. E

Hypothyroidism stimulates an increase in the production of thyrotropin releasing hormone (TRH) from the hypothalamus via a feedback loop. Although the primary role of TRH is to stimulate TSH release, it also stimulates the release of prolactin from the anterior pituitary gland, resulting in hyperprolactinaemia. Dopamine has an inhibitory effect on the release of prolactin. Prolactin stimulates development of the mammary glands and the production of milk towards the end of pregnancy. Causes of hyperprolactinaemia include pregnancy, medications that inhibit dopamine (e.g. antipsychotics), hypothyroidism and benign pituitary tumours. Hyperprolactinaemia leads to the inhibition of the release of gonadotrophin-releasing hormone (GnRH) from the hypothalamus, thereby inhibiting the production of FSH and LH from the anterior pituitary. This results in hypogonadism which manifests as amenorrhoea, erectile dysfunction and loss of libido. Women may also experience galactorrhoea.

Paper 10

Questions

1. An 18-year-old student is brought to see his GP by his mother. Since returning from university 2 days ago, he has become drowsy and has developed a fever. He has also vomited three times. On examination, the patient complains of pain when the GP flexes his hip and extends his knee, and a non-blanching rash is seen on his trunk. What should the GP do next?

   A Reassure and discharge
   B Administer IV or IM benzylpenicillin and call an ambulance
   C Administer IV dexamethasone and call an ambulance
   D Prescribe oral benzylpenicillin and arrange a follow up appointment
   E Prescribe oral dexamethasone and arrange a follow up appointment

2. A 24-year-old man presents to the outpatient clinic with a 3-month history of lower abdominal pain and bloody diarrhoea. He often defecates more than four times per day and sometimes does not feel completely empty afterwards. On examination, his fingers are clubbed and a large irregular ulcer is found on his left shin. What is the most likely diagnosis?

    A Irritable bowel syndrome
    B Gastroenteritis
    C Crohn's disease
    D Ulcerative colitis
    E Coeliac disease

3. Which joint is most commonly affected in gout?

    A 1st metacarpophalangeal joint
    B 1st metatarsophalangel joint
    C 1st tarsometatarsal joint
    D 1st interphalangeal joint
    E Talonavicular joint

4. A 10-year-old boy is brought to the respiratory clinic by his mother. Since he was very young, he has suffered from recurrent infections and has been hospitalized many times. As he has frequently moved country, a formal diagnosis has never been made. In the past 6 months, he has become increasingly breathless and has experienced a chronic cough, productive of large volumes of purulent sputum. A chest X-ray is performed revealing widespread bronchiectasis, and situs inversus. What is the most likely diagnosis?

    A Cystic fibrosis
    B Young's syndrome
    C Kartagener's syndrome
    D Caplan's syndrome
    E α_1 antitrypsin deficiency

5. Which system is used to stage Hodgkin's lymphoma?

    A Ann Arbor
    B Gleason
    C Dukes'
    D Rai and Binet
    E Breslow

6. A 63-year-old woman presents with a moist, shallow ulcer just superior to the medial malleolus of her left foot. It is diagnosed as a venous ulcer. Which of the following features is not associated with venous ulcers?

    A Varicose veins
    B Calloused edges
    C Stasis eczema
    D Haemosiderin deposition
    E Lipodermatosclerosis

7. Which of these conditions does not typically cause eye signs?

    A Ulcerative colitis
    B Crohn's disease
    C Ankylosing spondylitis
    D Reactive arthritis
    E Cervical spondylosis

8. Whilst enjoying a drink in a bar with some friends, a 36-year-old woman feels a sudden sensation of tingling in her ring finger which spreads to the rest of her hand over a couple of seconds. She only feels the sensation in her right hand and she maintains awareness throughout the episode, which lasts less than a minute. What type of seizure is this describing?

    A Absence
    B Simple partial
    C Complex partial
    D Myoclonic
    E Atonic

9. An 82-year-old lady has been in hospital for 4 weeks due to a hip fracture that she sustained after falling at home. Due to her immobility, a pressure sore has developed on the heel of her right foot. There

is an intact fluid-filled blister measuring 3 inches in diameter. The ulcer is superficial and there is no subcutaneous tissue visible. According to the EPUAP, what grade of severity is this pressure ulcer?

A Grade 1
B Grade 2
C Grade 3
D Grade 4
E Ungradable

10. What is the most common cause of encephalitis in the UK?

A Herpes simplex virus
B Syphilis
C EBV
D Varicella zoster virus
E Coxsackie virus

11. A 49-year-old bird keeper has become more and more breathless over the last 6 months. She used to be able to easily complete her daily dog walk, however, recently, she found that she has to take more breaks to catch her breath. She has also had a dry cough. Examination reveals fine inspiratory crackles and a chest X-ray shows reticulo-nodular shadowing. What is the most likely diagnosis?

A Extrinsic allergic alveolitis
B COPD
C Pneumoconiosis
D Aspergillosis
E Asbestosis

12. A 64-year-old man has been referred for an outpatient appointment with the urology department. Over the past 5 months, he has been urinating around 10–12 times per day. He often takes several minutes to start urinating and his stream is much weaker than it used to be. Once he has finished, he does not feel 'completely empty' and finds

that he 'leaks a little bit' as well. Digital rectal examination reveals a smoothly enlarged prostate gland with a palpable midline sulcus. A diagnosis of benign prostatic hyperplasia is made. He is eager to avoid surgery if possible. Which treatment would be best for him?

    A Oxybutynin
    B Solifenacin
    C Tamsulosin
    D Nitrofurantoin
    E Co-trimoxazole

13. A 53-year-old lady has been feeling increasingly short of breath over the past 6 months. She adds that she always feels very tired and has, more recently, experienced a tingling sensation in both hands. Neurological examination reveals a sensory neuropathy affecting only the hands and feet. What is the most likely cause of her symptoms?

    A Iron deficiency anaemia
    B Anaemia of chronic disease
    C Folic acid deficiency
    D Vitamin B12 deficiency
    E Thalassemia trait

14. A 33-year-old female with SLE presents to the fertility clinic complaining of repeated miscarriages. She has been desperately trying to start a family but has unfortunately suffered three miscarriages over the last 7 years. Her past medical history includes an appendicectomy (aged 12) and two DVTs. Given the likely diagnosis, which of the following antibodies is associated with this disease?

    A Anti-CCP antibody
    B Anti-Jo-1 antibody
    C Anti-centromere antibody
    D Anti-cardiolipin antibody
    E Anti-smooth muscle antibody

15. Which of the following is not associated with infective endocarditis?

   A Clubbing
   B Janeway lesions
   C Rose spots
   D New pansystolic murmur
   E Splinter haemorrhages

16. A 43-year-old woman presents with a 'rather embarrassing' problem. Since the birth of her fourth child, 3 months ago, she has wet herself several times. She has noticed that whenever she laughs or coughs, a little bit of urine leaks out without her control. What is the name of this type of incontinence?

   A Functional incontinence
   B Stress incontinence
   C Urge incontinence
   D Overflow incontinence
   E Double incontinence

17. A 44-year-old man has been suffering from constant, nagging head-aches for the past 2 years. In this time, he has also noticed that his hands and feet appear to have grown as he has changed shoe size three times, and had to get his wedding ring cut off. He has been relatively healthy throughout his life except for undergoing surgery for carpal tunnel syndrome last year. What is the most likely diagnosis?

   A Cushing's disease
   B Acromegaly
   C Hypothyroidism
   D Gigantism
   E Prolactinoma

18. Which of the following is used to predict the severity of acute pancreatitis?

    A Alvarado score
    B Rockall score
    C Modified Glasgow score
    D Glasgow-Blatchford score
    E Child–Pugh score

19. A 31-year-old scuba diving instructor, living in the Maldives, had a seizure 3 days ago. He has no history of epilepsy, however, he has had persistent headaches over the past 5 months. He adds that the headaches are particularly bad when he goes to bed. On examination, a dark, irregular skin lesion is found on the back of his neck. An MRI scan shows multiple lesions across both cerebral hemispheres. What is the most likely diagnosis?

    A Glioblastoma multiforme
    B Metastases
    C Neurofibromatosis type 1
    D Acoustic neuroma
    E Meningioma

20. Which of the following examination findings is not associated with COPD?

    A Use of accessory muscles
    B Breathing through pursed lips
    C Peripheral cyanosis
    D Clubbing
    E Bounding pulse

21. A 56-year-old man comes to A&E with a very swollen glans. He went to the toilet to urinate last night, however, once he had finished, he

was unable to replace his foreskin back over his glans. Since then, his glans has gradually become very painful and inflamed. What is the name of this condition?

    A Phimosis
    B Paraphimosis
    C Balanitis
    D Priapism
    E Peyronie's disease

22. A 59-year-old man presents to A&E with fatigue and shortness of breath that gets worse when lying down. He has also been coughing up pink, frothy sputum. An echocardiogram is performed, which shows aortic regurgitation. On closer inspection of the patient's hands, his nail beds appear to be pulsating. What is the name of this sign?

    A de Musset's sign
    B Quincke's sign
    C Traube's sign
    D Corrigan's sign
    E Becker's sign

23. A 61-year-old man attends an outpatient clinic appointment complaining of epigastric pain that gets better soon after eating. A urease breath test confirms the presence of *H. pylori*. A duodenal ulcer is suspected. What is the most appropriate management option?

    A 1 week of once daily omeprazole, amoxicillin and clarithromycin
    B 1 week of twice daily omeprazole, amoxicillin and clarithromycin
    C 1 week of once daily ranitidine, amoxicillin and clarithromycin
    D 1 week of twice daily ranitidine, amoxicillin and clarithromycin
    E 1 week of once daily omeprazole, ranitidine and amoxicillin

24. Which of the following is a major consequence of folate deficiency in pregnancy?

    A Incomplete limb development
    B Neural tube defects
    C Congenital cardiac abnormalities
    D High birth weight
    E Cleft palate

25. Which of the following is true about the target population group and frequency of breast cancer screening in the UK?

    A Women aged 35–65 every 3 years
    B Women aged 40–60 every 3 years
    C Women aged 40–70 every 5 years
    D Women aged 50–75 every 5 years
    E Women aged 50–70 every 3 years

26. A 46-year-old woman is brought to A&E complaining of severe right upper quadrant pain and a high fever with rigors. On examination, she is jaundiced, febrile and tachycardic. Vital Signs: RR = 24 breaths per minute, HR = 112 bpm, Temp = 38.9°C.

    A full blood count is requested:

    Hb = 142 g/L (115–160)
    WBC = 14.7×10^9/L (4–11)
    Platelets = 370×10^9/L (150–400)
    She is diagnosed with ascending cholangitis and her disease is managed using 'The Sepsis Six' protocol. Which of the following is not part of 'The Sepsis Six'?

    A Give high-flow oxygen
    B Take blood smear
    C Give IV antibiotics
    D Measure urine output
    E Measure serum lactate

27. A 15-year-old girl is brought, by her mother, to see her GP. She is concerned that her daughter has been acting 'very weird' over the past few months. Having previously been quite shy and reserved, she has recently had several rude outbursts towards her parents. In addition, her performance at school has deteriorated. On examination, she appears slightly jaundiced. Closer inspection of her eyes using a slit-lamp shows dark rings around her iris. Given the most likely diagnosis, which of the following would you expect to see in the diagnostic work up?

    A Low serum caeruloplasmin
    B High serum copper
    C Low AST
    D Low ALP
    E High transferrin saturation

28. A 4-year-old boy, who has recently moved to the UK from Cameroon, has been suffering from frequent infections and breathing difficulties since he was born. His mother tells you that he always has a cough and regularly suffers from chest infections. He has also had some bowel problems — his stools are often loose and irregular. On examination, he appears small for his age, his fingers are clubbed and bilateral coarse crackles are heard on auscultation. Cystic fibrosis is suspected. Which investigation should be requested to confirm the diagnosis?

    A Chest X-ray
    B Sweat test
    C Faecal elastase
    D Sputum culture
    E Stool culture

29. Which of the following is not a risk factor for the formation of a DVT?

    A Factor V Leiden
    B Malignancy
    C Nephrotic syndrome

    D Antiphospholipid syndrome

    E Alcohol

30. A 77-year-old retired ship-builder presents to his GP complaining of a 4-month history of right-sided chest pain, shortness of breath and 4 kg of weight loss. A chest X-ray is requested, which shows an ill-defined mass at the right pleural margin. What is the most likely diagnosis?

    A Small cell lung cancer

    B Adenocarcinoma

    C Mesothelioma

    D Squamous cell lung cancer

    E Large cell lung cancer

Answers

1. B

A non-blanching rash, drowsiness, fever and vomiting are characteristics of meningitis. It is likely to be meningococcal meningitis because of the presence of the non-blanching rash. Meningitis spreads via respiratory secretions, so it is easily transmitted in close living quarters such as university halls. Other features of meningitis include headache, neck stiffness and photophobia. Pain on flexing the hip and extending the knee is referred to as 'Kernig's sign', a feature of meningeal irritation. As soon as bacterial meningitis is suspected in the community setting, IV or IM benzylpenicillin should be administered immediately and the patient should be urgently transferred to hospital for further antibiotic treatment. Dexamethasone may be used in secondary care to reduce cerebral oedema.

2. D

Out of the possible answers, gastroenteritis, Crohn's disease and ulcerative colitis (UC) are associated with bloody diarrhoea. Gastroenteritis tends to present acutely and does not have any extra-GI manifestations. Irritable bowel syndrome and coeliac disease tend to present with cramping abdominal pain, bloating, urgency and diarrhoea soon after consuming certain foods. Bloody diarrhoea and tenesmus are more commonly associated with an exacerbation of UC. Crohn's disease does not cause bloody diarrhoea as frequently as UC, and it is less likely to affect the rectum. The large ulcer on his shin is describing pyoderma gangrenosum, an ulcerative cutaneous condition associated with systemic diseases, such as IBD, rheumatoid arthritis, multiple myeloma and granulomatosis with polyangiitis.

3. B

Gout is a crystal arthropathy caused by the deposition of monosodium urate crystals in joints and soft tissues. It most commonly affects the metatarsophalangeal joint of the big toe — a condition called 'podagra'. Other manifestations of gout include tophi — depositions of urate crystals around tendons and on the pinna of the ear.

4. C

Primary ciliary dyskinesia (PCD) is a genetic disorder resulting in defective ciliary action in the respiratory tract. The defective cilia struggle to clear mucus from the lungs, resulting in recurrent respiratory tract infections, which, over time, lead to bronchiectasis. Patients with PCD also suffer from recurrent otitis media. The coordinated beating of the cilia play an important role in guiding the development of organs in their correct locations within the body. The defective cilia in PCD do not provide this guidance, and so there is a 50:50 chance of the organs developing on the wrong side of the body (situs inversus). Kartagener's syndrome is a combination of primary ciliary dyskinesia and situs inversus.

Caplan's syndrome refers to the combination of rheumatoid arthritis and pneumoconiosis. Young's syndrome is a rare condition featuring bronchiectasis, sinusitis and infertility.

5. A

  Ann Arbor — Hodgkin's and non-Hodgkin's lymphoma
  Gleason — Prostate cancer
  Dukes' — Colorectal cancer
  Rai and Binet — Chronic lymphocytic leukaemia
  Breslow — Melanoma

6. B

Venous ulcers are most commonly found just superior to the medial malleolus (also known as the gaiter area). The ulcers are usually large, shallow and relatively painless. They usually occur in patients with known venous insufficiency (i.e. varicose veins). Common associated features include haemosiderin deposition (appears as a dark area of skin around the ulcer), stasis eczema and lipodermatosclerosis (inflammation of subcutaneous fat). Severe lipodermatosclerosis can lead to an 'inverted champagne bottle' appearance of the legs. Calloused edges are a feature of neuropathic ulcers which typically occur in diabetic patients.

7. E

Several inflammatory conditions cause eye signs, in particular, HLA-B27 associated conditions (e.g. sarcoidosis, inflammatory bowel disease, ankylosing spondylitis and reactive arthritis). Cervical spondylosis is a degenerative process affecting the cervical vertebrae and intervertebral discs. It leads to compression of the spinal cord and spinal nerve roots resulting in neck pain and arm pain. It is not associated with causing eye signs.

8. B

This patient has experienced a simple partial seizure. Partial seizures, also commonly known as focal seizures, refer to seizures originating in a localised area of one cerebral hemisphere. Simple partial seizures (SPS) do not involve loss of consciousness, however, they often progress to become complex partial seizure (CPS). CPS affects a larger area of the brain than SPS and causes an impairment of consciousness. Both SPS and CPS can evolve into generalised seizures (partial seizures with secondary generalisation) by spreading to the other side of the brain.

In fact, this patient's seizure is a sub-type of SPS known as a Jacksonian march. This is caused by electrical activity that steadily travels through the primary motor cortex. This movement of electrical activity causes a tingling sensation to 'march' across a region of the body from one group of distal muscles to another. In this patient's case, this began in her finger and then travelled up her hand. These 'march' like sensations are often accompanied by involuntary movements (automatisms), such as lip smacking or tapping, muscle cramping, hallucinations and head turning.

9. B

Pressure ulcers tend to form over bony prominences when prolonged pressure on the area completely or partially obstructs the blood flow to the tissues, leading to ischaemia and necrosis. Risk factors include immobility, malnourishment, vascular diseases (e.g. atherosclerosis), reduced sensation (e.g. paralysis), wet skin and old age. The European Pressure

Ulcer Advisory Panel (EPUAP) has devised a grading system to rate the severity of pressure ulcers. It consists of four grades, starting from grade 1 (the least severe).

- **Grade 1**: intact skin with non-blanching erythema. May be painful or itchy.
- **Grade 2**: partial thickness loss of dermis presenting as a shallow open ulcer with a red wound bed, without slough. May also present as an intact blister without bruising.
- **Grade 3**: full thickness skin loss. Subcutaneous tissue may be visible but bone, tendon and muscle are not. Slough may be present. Undermining and tunneling may occur.
- **Grade 4**: full thickness tissue loss with exposed bone, tendon and muscle. Slough or eschar may be present and undermining and tunneling usually present.

10. A

Encephalitis is an infection of the brain parenchyma that presents with reduced consciousness, focal neurology or seizures on the background of infectious symptoms such as lymphadenopathy and fever. Encephalitis is usually viral, with the most common cause being herpes simplex virus. Other viral causes include varicella zoster virus, EBV and Coxsackie virus. There are also several non-viral causes such as syphilis, toxoplasmosis and listeria.

11. A

Gradually worsening shortness of breath and a dry cough, with examination and imaging revealing fine inspiratory crackles and reticulo-nodular shadowing, is strongly suggestive of interstitial lung disease. Interstitial lung disease is a broad term used to describe an array of diseases that affect the lung parenchyma. The patient's occupation, bird-keeping, is an important clue. It suggests that she has had chronic exposure to bird droppings which can lead to a hypersensitivity reaction known as extrinsic allergic alveolitis (EAA). EAA can be acute, causing symptoms that resemble atypical pneumonia, or it can be chronic, resulting in pulmonary fibrosis. In summary, EAA is a hypersensitivity reaction to organic dusts (e.g. bird droppings).

Pneumoconiosis is a similar condition resulting in pulmonary fibrosis due to chronic inhalation of inorganic dusts (e.g. coal dust). Asbestosis is a type of pneumoconiosis, in which pulmonary fibrosis is caused by chronic exposure to asbestos. Aspergillosis is caused by an *Aspergillus fumigatus* infection. It does not tend to cause extensive pulmonary fibrosis. COPD usually occurs in patients with an extensive smoking history and it will usually present with gradually worsening shortness of breath with a cough productive of clear sputum.

12. C

Benign prostatic hyperplasia (BPH) is a very common condition caused by hyperplasia of the periurethral zone of the prostate gland. It leads to frequency, urgency and obstructive symptoms such as hesitancy, poor stream and incomplete voiding. BPH can be treated medically using α-blockers, such as tamsulosin, which relaxes the smooth muscle around the bladder neck and prostate, hence reducing the resistance to urinary outflow. 5α-reductase inhibitors, such as finasteride, can also be used — they inhibit the conversion of testosterone to dihydrotestosterone (a potent androgen) and reduces prostate volume.

Oxybutynin and Solifenacin are anticholinergics used to treat urinary incontinence. Nitrofurantoin and co-trimoxazole are antibiotics often used to treat UTIs.

13. D

Vitamin B12 deficiency is an important cause of megaloblastic anaemia. The body usually stores a large amount of vitamin B12 in the liver, so it takes several years to develop B12 deficiency. It is found in meat and other animal products. Once ingested, B12 binds to intrinsic factor (produced by the gastric parietal cells), forming a complex that is then absorbed in the terminal ileum. B12 is required to produce thymidine, a crucial building block of DNA, so B12 deficiency leads to impaired DNA production and, therefore, impaired red blood cell production. Causes of B12 deficiency include dietary deficiency, pernicious anaemia (lack of intrinsic factor due to autoimmune atrophic gastritis), terminal ileal resection and Crohn's disease. B12 deficiency causes the typical anaemic symptoms of pallor, shortness of breath and fatigue but it can also cause neurological symptoms (e.g. paraesthesia, peripheral neuropathy) — because vitamin B12 is required to maintain the integrity of the nervous system. It may also cause psychiatric symptoms such as depression and psychosis. The presence of neurological symptoms is distinctive of vitamin B12 deficiency anaemia. All the other options can cause anaemia, however, they will not cause peripheral neuropathy.

14. D

Antiphospholipid syndrome is a disease that is associated with four main features: thrombophilia (recurrent DVT/PE), livedo reticularis (mottled appearance of the skin), obstetric issues (recurrent miscarriage), and thrombocytopaenia. Antiphospholipid syndrome can occur on its own, or it can occur in association with SLE. The main antibodies tested in the diagnosis of antiphospholipid syndrome are lupus anticoagulant and anti-cardiolipin antibodies.

Other options and associations:

Anti-CCP — Rheumatoid Arthritis
Anti-Jo-1 — Polymyositis
Anti-Centromere — Limited Cutaneous Systemic Sclerosis
Anti-Smooth Muscle — Autoimmune Hepatitis

15. C

Infective endocarditis is an infection of structures within the heart (usually the valves). It leads to the formation of bacterial vegetations on heart valves leading to the destruction of these valves. Patients presenting with a new-onset heart murmur and a fever should be regarded as having infective endocarditis until proven otherwise. The major risk factors are recent dental surgery (portal of entry for *S. viridans*) and IV drug use. Signs of infective endocarditis include fever, tachycardia, clubbing, Janeway lesions, Osler's nodes, Roth spots on the retina, new murmurs and splinter haemorrhages. Rose spots are small red macules that appear on the torso of some patients with typhoid fever.

16. B

Urinary incontinence refers to the lack of voluntary control over urination. There are three main types: functional, stress and urge. Stress incontinence is when a small volume of urine leaks from an incompetent sphincter, whenever there is an increase in intra-abdominal pressure (e.g. laughing and coughing). It is common in pregnant women and following childbirth. It is also associated with pelvic floor weakness (e.g. uterine prolapse). Urge incontinence is when the feeling of needing to urinate is rapidly followed by uncontrollable urination. It results from detrusor overactivity (due to a neurological problem or an intrinsic problem with the detrusor muscle). Triggers include the cold, arriving at home and the sound of running water. Functional incontinence is when patients are unable to find a toilet before urinating. It occurs because of factors like immobility or being in unfamiliar surroundings rather than due to physiological dysfunction.

Overflow incontinence is the involuntary release of urine from a full bladder. This occurs in patients with bladder outflow obstruction or detrusor weakness. Double incontinence refers to the combination of faecal and urinary incontinence associated with neurological disorders such as multiple sclerosis and Alzheimer's disease.

17. B

Acromegaly is a disease caused by excessive production of growth hormone (GH) in adults — usually due to a GH-secreting pituitary adenoma. Excess GH before puberty is referred to as gigantism. The symptoms manifest very gradually over a period of years. Patients may notice that their hands and feet have grown, with an increase in shoe size and tightening rings being a common feature in SBAs. The space-occupying effects of a pituitary adenoma in acromegaly can lead to a chronic headache. The adenoma can also compress the optic chiasm leading to bitemporal hemianopia. The excess circulating GH can stimulate soft tissue growth in the wrists, resulting in carpal tunnel syndrome. Acromegaly patients also tend to have very distinctive facial features including prominent supraorbital ridges, thick lips, large tongue and prognathism.

18. C

The modified Glasgow score is used to predict the severity of acute pancreatitis and the resulting mortality. It consists of eight criteria which can be remembered using the mnemonic **PANCREAS**:

- **P**aO$_2$ < 7.9 kPa
- **A**ge > 55 years
- **N**eutrophilia (WCC > 15 × 10^9/L)
- **C**alcium < 2 mmol
- **R**enal function (urea > 16 mmol)
- **E**nzymes (LDH > 600 U/L or AST > 200 U/L)
- **A**lbumin < 32 g/L
- **S**ugar > 10 mmol

A score of 3 or more indicates severe pancreatitis.

The Alvarado score is used in the diagnosis of appendicitis. The Glasgow-Blatchford score is used to assess whether patients with upper GI bleeds should be managed as outpatients or should receive urgent intervention. Similarly, the Rockall score is used to predict the risk of re-bleeding and mortality in patients with upper GI bleeds. The Child–Pugh score is used to predict the prognosis of patients with cirrhosis.

19. B

This is a bit of a trick question because the presence of neurological symptoms with skin lesions makes many people carelessly jump to a diagnosis of neurofibromatosis. This patient has had persistent headaches for 5 months that are worse when he goes to bed (i.e. lies down) — this is a classic feature of space-occupying brain lesions. Brain tumours are also known to present with symptoms of neurological dysfunction such as seizures, paraesthesia and changes in speech, vision and hearing. Most brain tumours are caused by metastatic spread of cancer from elsewhere in the body. In this patient, the sinister skin lesion on the back of his neck is likely to be a melanoma that has metastasised to his brain. Furthermore, his job as a scuba diving instructor in the Maldives involves sun exposure and a high risk of developing skin cancer.

The presence of multiple brain tumours makes this less likely to be glioblastoma multiforme or meningioma, which tend to occur as single discrete lesions. Acoustic neuromas tend to be unilateral, however, bilateral acoustic neuromas are a feature of neurofibromatosis type 2. Neurofibromatosis type 1 tends to cause fewer central nervous system lesions and has more widespread peripheral features, such as neurofibromas, café au lait macules (>5 is significant), axillary freckling, Lisch nodules and spinal scoliosis. The lesion described in this SBA sounds more like a melanoma than a cutaneous feature of neurofibromatosis.

20. D

The main respiratory causes of clubbing are lung cancer, interstitial lung disease and chronic suppurative lung disease (e.g. empyema, bronchiectasis, cystic fibrosis). COPD is not a cause of finger clubbing.

Patients with severe COPD may use their accessory muscles (e.g. sternocleidomastoid) when breathing to assist elevation of the rib cage during inspiration. Patients may also breathe through pursed lips, which keeps the airways open for longer and reduces the work of breathing. In addition, COPD can lead to peripheral cyanosis (due to low oxygen saturation) and a bounding pulse (due to carbon dioxide retention).

21. B

Paraphimosis is a urological emergency that occurs when a tight foreskin is retracted and then cannot be replaced back over the glans. The tight foreskin prevents venous return from the tip of the glans, leading to oedema and, sometimes, ischaemia of the glans. It can be iatrogenic — when the foreskin is not replaced after catheterization. It is usually treated by manually applying pressure to the glans. Lidocaine gel may be used to help deal with the pain.

Phimosis is when a tight foreskin occludes the meatus. It can lead to recurrent infections and ballooning. Balanitis is inflammation of the foreskin and glans. Diabetics and young children with tight foreskins are at increased risk. Priapism is a persistent and painful erection that is associated with haematological disorders — most commonly sickle cell disease. Peyronie's disease refers to the growth of fibrous plaques in the soft tissue of the penis. This leads to pain, abnormal curvature of the penis and erectile dysfunction.

22. B

Aortic regurgitation (AR) is a valve defect characterised by the reflux of blood from the aorta into the left ventricle during diastole. There are several causes of AR including bicuspid aortic valve, infective endocarditis and rheumatic fever. AR can lead to heart failure, and, hence, presents with symptoms such as dyspnoea, orthopnoea and a cough productive of pink, frothy sputum. The main clinical signs of AR are a collapsing ('water-hammer') pulse, wide pulse pressure and an early diastolic murmur. However, AR is renowned for having a multitude of eponymous signs — here are some of them:

Quincke's Sign — visible pulsation on the nail beds
De Musset's Sign — head nodding in time with the pulse
Traube's Sign — 'pistol-shot' (loud systolic and diastolic sounds) heard over the femoral artery
Corrigan's Sign — visible pulsation in the neck
Becker's Sign — visible pulsation of the pupils and retinal arteries.

23. B

Duodenal ulcers are four times more common than gastric ulcers and *H. pylori* is implicated in 90% of duodenal ulcers and 80% of gastric ulcers. *H. pylori* is eradicated using triple therapy: A 1 week treatment regimen consisting of a PPI (e.g. omeprazole) and two antibiotics (most commonly amoxicillin and clarithromycin or clarithromycin and metronidazole) — each drug is taken twice daily. Triple therapy is effective in 80–85% of cases. If this fails, then second-line therapy involves using a different combination of antibiotics or adding a bismuth compound (quadruple therapy).

24. B

Neural tube defects are caused by a failure of closure of the neural tube during intrauterine development. There are two main types — spina bifida (affecting the spinal cord) and anencephaly (affecting the brain). To prevent neural tube defects, pregnant women are given folic acid supplements. This has led to a decrease in the prevalence of neural tube defects. Folic acid deficiency is also associated with low birth weight.

25. E

Breast cancer screening, using mammography, in the UK is currently offered to women aged 50–70 years. They will be invited for a check-up every 3 years.

26. B

Sepsis is defined as systemic inflammatory response syndrome (SIRS) with a suspected or confirmed infectious cause. SIRS is defined by the following parameters: temperature $> 38°C$ or $< 36°C$; respiratory rate > 20/min or $PaCO_2 < 4.3$ kPa; heart rate > 90 bpm; white cell count $> 12,000$ cells/mm^3 or < 4000 cells/mm^3. The sepsis six is a protocol used in the initial management of sepsis and it can be remembered as '3 in and 3 out' (i.e. you are taking three samples from the patient, and you are giving the patient three interventions).

The Sepsis Six

1. **IN** – Give high flow oxygen
2. **OUT** – Take blood cultures
3. **IN** – Give empirical IV antibiotics
4. **IN** – Give an IV fluid challenge
5. **OUT** – Measure serum lactate and haemoglobin
6. **OUT** – Measure urine output.

27. A

Wilson's disease is an autosomal recessive disease caused by impaired biliary copper excretion, which leads to an accumulation of copper in various tissues (most notably, the liver and the brain). Wilson's disease usually presents in children and young adults with symptoms of liver dysfunction (e.g. jaundice, easy bruising, variceal bleeding) or neuropsychiatric dysfunction (e.g. personality change, dysarthria, dyskinesia). Despite being a very rare disease, it is well-known amongst medical students because of its clinical hallmark — dark concentric rings around the edge of the iris called 'Kayser–Fleischer rings'. Biochemically, Wilson's disease can be confusing because the parameters change in a somewhat paradoxical way. Commit the following to memory.

Wilson's disease causes: *Low* serum caeruloplasmin + *Low* serum copper.

Wilson's disease leads to hepatitis and cirrhosis, which results in elevated liver enzymes (e.g. AST, ALT, ALP). A high transferrin saturation is seen in haemochromatosis.

28. B

Cystic fibrosis (CF) is an autosomal recessive condition caused by a mutation in a chloride ion channel (CFTR). This leads to the production of defective chloride ion channels and abnormally thick secretions. Thick mucus in the respiratory tract can be difficult for the cilia to clear, so it can accumulate and is prone to infection. This can lead to respiratory symptoms such as recurrent infections, bronchiectasis, cough and wheeze. Abnormally thick pancreatic secretions may lead to pancreatic insufficiency (manifesting as diabetes mellitus and steatorrhoea). CF patients are also at increased risk of developing gallstones. Clinical signs of CF include clubbing, cyanosis and bilateral coarse crackles. A sweat test measures the chloride concentration of the patient's sweat. If the chloride concentration is >60 mmol/L, a diagnosis of CF is likely. Faecal elastase can be used to assess the extent of pancreatic exocrine insufficiency in CF.

29. E

Low to moderate alcohol consumption is associated with a decreased risk of DVTs. Virchow's triad describes the three factors that contribute to the formation of venous thromboses. All DVT risk factors will affect at least one of the components of the triad.

1. **Stasis**: immobility, surgery, varicose veins, polycythaemia, venous obstruction (from pregnancy, tumour or obesity)
2. **Endothelial injury**: smoking, trauma, surgery, vascular catheterisation and hypertension
3. **Hypercoagulability**: malignancy, pregnancy, hormone therapy, combined oral contraceptive pill, nephrotic syndrome, inflammatory bowel disease, obesity, Factor V Leiden, protein C or S deficiency and antiphospholipid syndrome.

30. C

A mesothelioma is a malignant tumour of the mesothelial cells, which usually occurs in the pleura but can be found in other sites (e.g. peritoneum, pericardium). It is a very aggressive tumour that has a poor prognosis. Mesothelioma is strongly related to asbestos exposure, which is most common amongst ship-builders, carpenters, factory workers and other occupations that involve working in old buildings containing asbestos. It usually presents with shortness of breath, chest pain and weight loss. A chest X-ray will show a mass along the pleura.

Lung cancer can be divided into small cell lung cancer and non-small cell lung cancer (NSCLC). Small cell lung cancer is most common amongst smokers and has a poorer prognosis than NSCLC, however, it only accounts for 20% of all lung cancers. The main subtypes of NSCLC are adenocarcinoma, squamous cell carcinoma and large cell carcinoma.

Index

D

deep vein thrombosis (DVT), 26, 227, 260
delirium tremens, 106
dementia, 44, 109
de Quervain's thyroiditis, 77
dermatitis herpetiformis, 67, 206
desmopressin, 22
DEXA scan, 17
diabetes insipidus (DI), 21, 234
diabetes mellitus, 19, 50, 155, 159
diabetic retinopathy, 18
dialysis, 187
digital rectal examination (DRE), 50
disseminated intravascular coagulation (DIC), 23, 183
diverticulitis, 79, 129
Dressler's syndrome, 25

E

E. coli, 23, 149, 182, 200, 207, 231
eczema, 96–97
encephalitis, 251
epididymal cyst, 73, 105
epilepsy, 101, 151, 204, 250
Epstein–Barr virus (EBV), 26, 126, 176
erythema multiforme, 107
erythema nodosum, 69, 202, 206
erythrocyte sedimentation rate (ESR), 39, 68, 131, 152, 154, 226, 230

F

faecal elastase, 15
fasting blood glucose, 50
Felty's syndrome, 133

fibroadenoma, 77–78, 155, 178, 226
fibrocystic disease, 178

G

gallstones, 123, 203
gastric cancer, 51
gastroenteritis, 46, 67, 148, 200, 206, 248
gastro-oesophageal reflux disease (GORD), 95, 160, 187
Gilbert's syndrome, 203
glandular fever (*see* infectious mononucleosis), 26
glasgow coma scale (GCS), 13, 212
glomerulonephritis, 14, 19, 95, 154, 156, 211, 224, 230
gonorrhoea, 39
Goodpasture's syndrome, 99, 154, 156
gout, 49, 201, 248
GRACE score, 18, 234
granulomatosis with polyangiitis (GPA), 99, 154
Graves' disease, 77, 180
Guillain–Barré syndrome (GBS), 48, 19, 182, 229
gynaecomastia, 160

H

haemochromatosis, 225
haemolytic uraemic syndrome (HUS), 23
haemophilia, 128
haemorrhoids, 25, 132
heart failure, 68, 127, 133, 152, 185, 202, 208, 210, 224, 230
helicobacter pylori, 75
hemianopia, 102, 226